Systematic Treatment of Persistent Psychosis (STOPP):

A psychological approach to facilitating recovery in young people with first-episode psychosis

Systematic Treatment of Persistent Psychosis (STOPP):

A psychological approach to facilitating recovery in young people with first-episode psychosis

Tanya Herrmann-Doig BA,
Grad Dip App Child Psych, MPsych (Clin), MAPS
Research Fellow in the Department of Psychiatry,
University of Melbourne
Parkville, Australia

Dana Maude BSc (Hons), MPsych (Clin), MAPS
Consultant Clinical Psychologist
Early Psychosis Prevention and Intervention Centre (EPPIC)/ Mental Health Services for Kids and Youth (MH-SKY),

Jane Edwards BA (Hons),
MA (Clin Psych), PhD, MAPS
Deputy Clinical Director
Early Psychosis Prevention and Intervention Centre (EPPIC)/ Mental Health Services for Kids and Youth (MH-SKY), and Fellow of the Departments of Psychiatry and Psychology,
University of Melbourne, Parkville, Australia

MARTIN DUNITZ

First published in the United Kingdom in 2003
by Martin Dunitz, Taylor & Francis Group plc, 11 New Fetter Lane, London EC4P 4EE

Tel.: +44 (0) 20 7583 9855
Fax.: +44 (0) 20 7842 2298
E-mail: info@dunitz.co.uk
Website: http://www.dunitz.co.uk

A CIP record for this book is available from the British Library.

ISBN 1 84184 224 9

Distributed in the USA by
Fulfilment Center
Taylor & Francis
10650 Tobben Drive
Independence, KY 41051, USA
Toll Free Tel.: +1 800 634 7064
E-mail: taylorandfrancis@thomsonlearning.com

Distributed in Canada by
Taylor & Francis
74 Rolark Drive
Scarborough, Ontario M1R 4G2, Canada
Toll Free Tel.: +1 877 226 2237
E-mail: tal_fran@istar.ca

Distributed in Australia and New Zealand by
Blackwell Publishing Asia
550 Swanston Street
Carlton
Victoria 3053, Australia
Tel.: +61 (0) 393470300
Website: www.blackwellpublishingasia.com

Distributed in the rest of the world by
Thomson Publishing Services
Cheriton House
North Way
Andover, Hampshire SP10 5BE, UK
Tel.: +44 (0)1264 332424
E-mail: salesorder.tandf@
thomsonpublishingservices.co.uk

Distributed in the rest of the world by:
Thomson Publishing Services
Cheriton House
North Way
Andover, Hampshire SP10 5BE, UK

Composition by Wearset Ltd, Boldon, Tyne & Wear.
Printed and bound in Great Britain by The Cromwell Press

Contents

About the authors vii

Forewords ix

Preface xii

Acknowledgements xv

1. Introduction 1
2. Psychological interventions for psychotic disorders 7
3. Negotiating the therapeutic process 13
4. Phase 1: developing a collaborative working relationship 19
5. Phase 2. Exploring and coping with psychosis 33
6. Phase 3: strengthening the capacity to relate to others 51
7. Phase 4: finishing and moving on 63

References 73

Appendix I 79

Appendix II 85

Index 93

Permission

The case material of 'Fiona' (see Chapters 5 and 6) has been adapted and reproduced with permission of the American Psychiatric Association from Edwards J, Maude D, Herrmann-Doig T, Wong L, Cocks J et al (2002b).

About the authors

Tanya Herrmann-Doig BA, Grad Dip App Child Psych, MPsych (Clin), MAPS, a Research Fellow in the Department of Psychiatry, University of Melbourne, is a STOPP therapist for the Recovery Plus Project. Prior to undertaking the role of Recovery Plus Project co-ordinator (1998–2000) she worked as a research therapist in an intervention study concerning early psychosis and suicide prevention.

Dana Maude BSc (Hons), MPsych (Clin), MAPS, is currently employed by a statewide service which provides consultation regarding individuals with severe personality disorders. She has a part time private practice and acts as a consultant to the Recovery Plus Project. Dana worked as clinical psychologist in the assessment and outpatient teams at the Early Psychosis Prevention and Intervention Centre (EPPIC) for 5 years before undertaking the role of Recovery Plus Project co-ordinator (1996–1998).

Jane Edwards BA (Hons), MA (Clin Psych), PhD, MAPS, is the Deputy Clinical Director of EPPIC/Mental Health Services for Kids and Youth (MH-SKY) and Fellow of the Departments of Psychiatry and Psychology, University of

Melbourne. She is the key investigator of the Recovery Plus Project. Jane has worked with young people experiencing early psychosis since 1985 and recently published a book, co-authored with Patrick McGorry, entitled *Implementing Early Intervention in Psychosis: A Guide to Establishing Early Psychosis Services* (Martin Dunitz, 2002).

Forewords

The therapist's skill and art lie in keeping things simple enough so that something can happen.

HS Sullivan: The Psychiatric Interview, p 216, 1954.

At the rate that new clinical and scientific knowledge concerning schizophrenia is becoming available, keeping things simple is not so easy. Current views of the cause of schizophrenia are grounded in a stress-vulnerability model that posits a complex interplay of genetic and environmental risk factors operating from intrauterine life onward. A developmental perspective focuses attention on the psychobiological antecedents of schizophrenia, in the form of aberrations in the developing central nervous system and the subjective and interpersonal self. Consequently, schizophrenia is seen as a phasic illness that includes premorbid, prodromal, acute and post-acute phases along with periods of progression, relapse, remission, clinical plateaus and recoveries. Finally, because of substantial variability in both the illness and those afflicted with it, there is no 'typical case' of schizophrenia. Individuals carrying this diagnosis differ markedly from each other in pre-illness functioning and abilities, age and type of illness onset, severity of positive, negative and cognitive symptoms, illness course and level of long-term disability or recovery. Given these individual differences, it is clear that where treatment is concerned, one size does not fit all.

Clinicians and investigators at the University of Melbourne's *Early Psychosis Prevention and Intervention Centre (EPPIC)* are leaders in elaborating the clinical implications of modern scientific conceptions of schizophrenia and other psychoses. Their groundbreaking work during the 1990s in establishing clinical services for individuals in the prodromal and early acute phase of psychosis, described in the monograph *Implementing Early Intervention in Psychosis: A Guide to Establishing Early Psychosis Services,* has catalyzed widespread interest in the prospect of favorably altering the long-term course of this illness through early detection and treatment. This simple, but powerful idea has ignited renewed optimism and a keen interest in reassessing public health approaches to psychoses throughout the world.

Research indicates that with appropriate and timely treatment most patients achieve substantial remission of symptoms following a first episode of psychosis. But what of those young people who do not fully respond? Those who experience persistent symptoms of psychosis despite adequate psychosocial support and medications?

Developed in the context of the Melbourne Early Psychosis Service, STOPP (Systematic Treatment of Persistent Psychosis) is a treatment developed for young people, in the early post-acute phase of a first psychotic episode who are experiencing persistent symptoms or what the authors call 'prolonged recovery'. Designed as a time-limited treatment added on to usual supportive care, the goal of STOPP is to prevent chronicity and treatment resistance by accelerating symptom remission and improving functioning. STOPP adapts techniques from effective cognitive therapies for persistent psychosis symptoms developed over the last decade in the United Kingdom to the special needs of young persons. Proceeding through phases of building relationships, learning coping skills, strengthening capacity to relate to others, and finishing and moving on, STOPP provides a coherent framework for enhancing outcome for patients at particularly high-risk for adverse outcomes. The results of a rigorous scientific evaluation of the therapy are in preparation as this book goes to press.

This STOPP manual is written by clinicians for clinicians and will be of immediate utility. Alongside prior work from the Melbourne group it succeeds in extracting simple and powerful principles for state of the art individualized management of a complex medical and psychosocial illness.

Wayne S Fenton
Bethesda, Maryland, USA

Evidence-based psychological treatments in psychosis are swiftly gaining recognition. Cognitive behaviour therapy has been shown to be effective in conjunction with routine care, in alleviating persistent symptoms of psychosis. Much of the recent evidence has come from people with treatment resistant chronic schizophrenia. However, the principles and methods are applicable, and the results potentially more important, in the subgroup of young people who suffer persistent symptoms in their first episode.

Over two thirds of young people in the first episode of psychosis will achieve remission in the space of 2–3 months, although styles of recovery vary. In addition, at least a quarter of individuals will carry on having disabling positive or negative symptoms. The Early Psychosis Prevention and Intervention Centre (EPPIC) has set up a ground breaking, modular approach to tackling problems which beset young people in first episode psychosis. These include existential problems to be expected in a cohort of individuals going through adolescence and early adult life, and clinical issues to do with the psychosis itself, as well as its aftermath.

Any individual going through EPPIC who has not made a substantial recovery by three months is comprehensively reviewed. STOPP, which is described here, is the psychological component of a wider treatment programme for early refractory symptoms in first episode psychosis. The handbook is clear, structured and practical. The rationale for, and delivery of, cognitive behaviour therapy in this client group is explained. Crucial stages of engagement, assessment, instigation of a collaborative approach and formulation to make sense of the problems and provide a rationale for future therapy, are set out. There is a focus on issues and complications which frequently arise, such as developmental issues, family problems, stigma, hopelessness, substance use and a potentially lasting traumatic nature of a psychotic episode itself.

By recognizing a particular clinical scenario of potentially lasting importance, refractory symptoms in the first episode, this book deserves to be read by all practitioners who deal with the increasing global focus on first episode psychosis.

Shôn Lewis
Withington Hospital, Manchester, UK

Preface

Systematic Treatment for Persistent Psychosis (STOPP) is a cognitively-orientated psychological therapy for young people with first episode psychosis who experience psychotic symptoms which persist beyond 3 months of initial treatment. The approach was developed at the Early Psychosis Prevention and Intervention Centre (EPPIC) in the context of a randomised controlled trial examining the relative and combined effectiveness of psychological and pharmacological approaches to prolonged recovery -'Recovery Plus'.

The onset of first episode psychosis occurs commonly in late adolescence or early adulthood, a critical stage of development in terms of psychological and social functioning. The consequences of failure to respond to standard treatment can be profound, including alienation from family and peers; and disruption of educational, vocational, and occupational goals. Chapter 1 discusses the potential benefits of comprehensive intervention in early psychosis, and flags the biopsychosocial context in which psychological therapies in first episode psychosis should be provided (Edwards et al 2002). Chapter 2 reviews the theoretical basis for psychological therapy with young people with psychosis, the strengths and limitations of cognitive-behavioural therapies with this target group, and the evolution of STOPP.

Chapters 3 to 7 outline the components of the intervention, describing practical issues to consider in implementation, the key therapy foci, and issues that commonly arise. STOPP is delivered in phases, commencing with the establishment of a collaborative working relationship, followed by exploring the experience of psychosis, developing skills for coping with symptoms, strengthening the capacity to relate to others, and then 'moving on'. The STOPP approach draws on empirically supported treatments for schizophrenia developed by researchers in the United Kingdom that have been well described (e.g. Kingdon & Turkington 1994; Fowler, Garety & Kuipers 1995; Chadwick, Birchwood & Trower 1996). In this text we focus on young people experiencing prolonged recovery from a first episode of psychosis, with the aim of *preventing* 'treatment resistance'. Strategies appropriate for *young people* in the *recent-onset phase* of illness are emphasised throughout.

Pilot work for STOPP was undertaken from 1993 and recruitment for the Recovery Plus study commenced in 1996. The three authors have been the STOPP therapists for all participants in the randomised controlled trial and worked psychologically with many others with enduring positive symptoms. Tanya Herrmann-Doig was the third therapist to join the team and rapidly learnt the STOPP approach through an intense period of supervision. Her ability to facilitate the translation of that knowledge into a written form, as part of her (then) new role as study co-ordinator, was outstanding. The strength of the manual is that Tanya represents the target audience – i.e. some experience with both cognitive-behavioural therapy and first episode psychosis *and* required to apply this knowledge to early treatment resistance as soon as possible. She has put pen to paper in a way that makes the work understandable, fresh, and real … providing a slant that may be have been out of reach for the more seasoned clinician/academic. Our aim has been to "outline sequenced interventions with sufficient specificity to allow them to be operationalized, taught, and measured, while retaining sufficient flexibility to accommodate patient heterogeneity" (Fenton 2000, p 67). The manuscript should prove immediately usable and workable, able to be read relatively quickly with suggestions for further reading if desired.

It should be noted that the rationale for focussing attention on this particular subgroup of young people with first episode psychosis partly arose from their exclusion from a cognitively oriented psychotherapy for early psychosis (COPE) which was evaluated at EPPIC between 1992 to 1999. COPE aims to facilitate adjustment of the person and prevention or alleviation of secondary morbidity in the wake of illness onset and was offered to individuals considered 'settled' by the treating clinicians (Jackson et al. 2001). The second and third authors of this manuscript were also COPE therapists. However, the separate and somewhat artificial separation of the two research projects allowed a concentrated effort on developing and articulating a psychological approach targeting prolonged recovery.

We are indebted to the young people who have agreed to work with us and hope that the sharing of experiences will encourage and empower.

Jane Edwards
Melbourne, Australia

Acknowledgements

We wish to thank the many EPPIC clinicians and young people with early psychosis who have contributed to the development of the ideas reflected in this book. Darryl Wade, John Gleeson, Olympia Athanasopoulos and Lisa Wong all made helpful comments on an earlier draft of the manuscript. Tony James provided constructive editorial assistance. Sue Leitinger assisted with the references and Bernie Cram designed the cover. The text was reviewed by Henry Jackson and Patrick McGorry (University of Melbourne, Parkville, Australia) and Jean Addington (University of Calgary, Alberta, Canada) – colleagues currently embarking on STOPP-like projects with first-episode patients and we are grateful for their suggestions. Our approach was influenced by the work of Kingdon and Turkington and we were honoured to receive and integrate the David Kingdon's thoughtful comments on the manuscript in the final stages of the endeavour. Writing was assisted by a Research Program and Project Grant from the Victorian Health Promotion Foundation (1999–2001).

1

Introduction

Background

The Systematic Treatment of Persistent Psychosis (STOPP) programme was developed at the Early Psychosis Prevention and Intervention Centre (EPPIC) in Melbourne, Victoria, Australia (McGorry et al 1996, Edwards and McGorry 2002, www.eppic.org.au). EPPIC is a comprehensive clinical and research service which aims to reduce the level of both primary and secondary morbidity in young people experiencing early psychosis through the dual strategy of identification of individuals at the earliest stage following onset of psychosis and provision of intensive phase-specific treatment for up to 18 months. It has a focus on empirically validated treatments, provides professional development through supervision and training and adheres to the Australian Clinical Guidelines for Early Psychosis (Edwards and McGorry 1998, Edwards et al in press).

The STOPP programme was developed to provide intensive interventions for young people experiencing first-episode psychosis who are at risk of developing a chronic course of illness. It was introduced within a broader treatment subprogramme of EPPIC, referred to as the Treatment

Resistant Early Assessment Team (TREAT), which detects patients experiencing a prolonged illness and implements interventions to facilitate recovery (Edwards et al 1998, 2002b, EPPIC 2002c).

Early intervention in psychosis

Recent years have seen the emergence of a special interest in the early phases of psychotic illness and the potential benefits of early intervention (McGlashan 1996, McGorry 1998). The association between the duration of untreated psychosis and outcome (see Norman and Malla 2001) has supported the notion that there may be a 'critical period' in which the ultimate course of the disorder is determined. Longer periods of untreated or active psychosis are related to slower and less complete recovery (Loebel et al 1992), higher relapse rates (Crow et al 1986) and lower levels of social and occupational functioning (Rabiner et al 1986, Wyatt 1991). This association is independent of the level of premorbid adjustment, the age and mode of illness onset and the severity of illness.

These findings suggest there is something about psychosis that is 'toxic' to the individual, and that an active process during periods of acute psychosis may be responsible for lasting disability (Loebel et al 1992, Wyatt et al 1989). In addition, it has been argued that morbidity which is secondary to the psychosis itself, such as the trauma of becoming unwell and entering into psychiatric care, or becoming depressed following the acute phase of illness, may play a significant role in the person's capacity to recover (Jackson et al 1999).

Attempts to improve the course of psychotic disorders must focus on:

- reducing the time between the onset of symptoms and the initiation of treatment
- accelerating remission from the first episode
- preventing relapse

Accelerating remission is the focus of the TREAT subprogramme at EPPIC. It is hoped that such interventions will ultimately reduce the establishment of treatment resistance.

Special needs of young people

The onset of a psychotic illness can have devastating effects at any age, but the long-term consequences may be particularly marked in young people. Jackson et al (1999) summarized the situation:

> *The effects of the psychosis on the self and development may be potentially cataclysmic, causing derailment, truncation, deflection or paralysis of the person's developmental trajectory. Psychosis has the potential to change or alter the person's usual way of construing themself, their environment and*

> *their future, and the devastation is further potentiated where the person is relatively young and developmentally 'immature'.* (p. 217)

Psychotic illness in a young person may be complicated by factors such as a high incidence of substance misuse, minimal prior experience with the health system (and particularly the mental health system), community-wide negative stereotypes of mental illness, fear of hospitalization and the use of denial as a protective strategy. In addition, young people often have a strong belief in their own invulnerability and poor acceptance of the fact that they are unwell and need treatment (EPPIC 2001).

The onset of psychosis in a young person is likely to interfere with the important tasks of adolescence and early adulthood. These tasks include individuating from the family, developing new interests and skills, discovering sexuality, forming and maintaining relationships and moving to further study or employment. Disruption caused by illness will often cause a young person to 'fall out of step' with their peers who are continuing to develop at the usual rate. Consequences include feelings of social isolation and demoralization and reduced potential for achievements in the future.

Persistence of symptoms after the onset of psychotic illness will further worsen the outlook for the young patient and exacerbate the difficulties caused by a disrupted developmental trajectory. Early detection of persisting symptoms and effective intervention should reduce the potential for damage.

Impact of substance misuse

Misuse of substances, particularly cannabis, is a common comorbid problem in first-episode psychosis (Edwards et al 2002a) and is relevant to a number of the case vignettes discussed in later chapters. The structure of the STOPP programme does not deal explicitly with substance misuse as a factor in the persistence of positive psychotic symptoms, but the issue cannot be ignored. It may be helpful to acknowledge some trends in current approaches to substance misuse (see Graham et al 2002), including the following:

- brief interventions are more effective than no intervention at all
- treatment should be matched to individuals' readiness to change
- harm minimization may be a more realistic aim than abstinence
- a first episode of psychosis can be a powerful motivator to change patterns of substance use

A cannabis-focused intervention has been developed at EPPIC for young people who continue to use cannabis after initial treatment for first-episode psychosis (EPPIC

2002b). The programme aims to develop an appreciation that cannabis use is potentially problematic in individuals with a psychotic illness and to develop a commitment to change cannabis use. Discussion of positive effects of cannabis (e.g. socialization and relaxation) as well as negative effects (e.g. exacerbation of psychosis, failure to respond to antipsychotic treatment, and financial, social and legal consequences) is required for a balanced assessment from which patients can draw their own conclusions and decide on future use or abstinence. The six phases of cannabis focused treatment are entry, commitment, goal setting, challenges, relapse prevention/lifestyle and maintenance. Resource materials include fact sheets (www.dhs.vic.gov.au/phd/hdev/cannabis/fact/contents.htm) and videos (www.abc.net.au/quantum/poison/marijuan/marijuan.htm).

Context of psychological treatment

Psychological intervention in the early phase of a psychotic disorder requires integration with the biological and social aspects of treatment (Edwards et al 2002b). Within the first 3 months of care, the biological interventions are likely to have involved a trial of at least one antipsychotic medication at therapeutic doses. Early social interventions may have included support and education to family, friends and places of employment or education and ensuring adequate financial support and housing. The psychological work in this phase may include developing a psychological understanding of the person, offering support and education and providing the opportunity to explore what has occurred (Jackson et al 2001).

If the young person's positive psychotic symptoms have not resolved within the first 3 months of treatment, we suggest a thorough review and consideration of more specialized biological, social, and psychological treatments (EPPIC 2002c). The biological input may include a review of antipsychotic medication and monitoring of compliance. The social component may involve more intensive family work and incorporation of group-based programmes. It is within this biopsychosocial context that specialized psychological interventions such as STOPP are best applied.

> A paper describing TREAT (Edwards et al 2002b) is reproduced in Appendix I.

Individuals and families at this phase of illness have a wide range of needs and STOPP therapy will need to be adapted accordingly. We have found it helpful to offer STOPP separately from case management where possible, allowing routine case management tasks to continue independently. It is important to spend time discussing the similarities and differences in the roles of the different people providing treatment and ensuring clear agreement and communication between the members of the team about the treatment plan.

An alternative approach is to incorporate a cognitive behavioural therapy approach into the case management role (see Turkington and Kingdon 2000). This may be practical provided that adequate resources are available, including additional staff time and an appropriate consulting room. At EPPIC this is sometimes provided as a first step, with the recognition that some patients will require a more concentrated cognitive behavioural approach at a later stage.

In either context, the STOPP worker requires adequate supervision from an experienced clinician. Skilled input is particularly important when working with a young person experiencing prolonged recovery *and* comorbid conditions on axes I–III of DSM-IV (American Psychiatric Association 1994) with which the therapist has had limited experience, such as body dysmorphic disorder (see Phillips 1996), intellectual disability or deafness.

A supportive clinical service will facilitate the implementation of STOPP. Features of the service to consider include:

- the service setting (is it age-appropriate? does it cater for the needs of young people?)
- transport issues (is the service easily accessible? can patients obtain transport to the service?)
- arrangement of appointments with the treating team (is the client overwhelmed by multiple contacts with service providers?)

In light of the disorganization often experienced by patients with psychosis, assistance with logistical barriers such as transport can improve participation in the programme. For example, this might include provision of public transport tickets or taxi vouchers. Home visits may be warranted, especially where the client is clearly unable to travel independently. Coordination of appointment times with other clinicians in the team is important in reducing the effort and potential confusion involved in attending the service. The possibility of 'scaling down' the frequency of other appointments while STOPP is in progress may need to be discussed with the treating team.

Evaluation of the STOPP programme

The STOPP programme is being evaluated as part of a randomized research trial at EPPIC. The Recovery Plus Project is one of the first studies to assess psychological treatments in patients with a prolonged recovery in early psychosis (Edwards et al 1998, 2002b).

A number of other researchers have examined the effectiveness of cognitive–behavioural interventions for enduring positive symptoms, but not specifically in first-episode patients (notably Kingdon and Turkington 1998, Garety et al 1994, 1997, Kuipers et al 1997, 1998, Tarrier 1992, Tarrier et al 1993a, b, 1998, 1999, 2000, Sensky et al 2000). Although these studies have some methodological limitations, 'the aggregate evidence suggests that under some circumstances cognitive–behavioural approaches may be effective in reducing frequency or severity of psychotic symptoms such as hallucinations and delusions' (Norman and Townsend 1999, p. 250). More recently a large multicentre trial has examined the potential of cognitive approaches to accelerating recovery in recent-onset psychosis (Haddock et al 1998a, Lewis et al 2001).

In the Recovery Plus Project, consecutive first-episode patients not achieving a predefined level of remission after the initial 12 weeks of standardized treatment are randomized into one of four groups for a further 12-week period:

- standard antipsychotic therapy and case management
- standard antipsychotic therapy, case management and STOPP therapy
- clozapine and case management
- clozapine, case management and STOPP therapy

Recruitment for the study commenced in September 1996 and continued until March 2002.

2

Psychological interventions for psychotic disorders

Theoretical framework

Introductions to recent texts have reviewed the role of individual psychological therapy with patients suffering from psychosis and have concluded that cognitive–behavioural therapies (CBT) are a valuable intervention (Martindale et al 2000, Perris and McGorry 1998). The sustained interest in these approaches has been attributed to factors such as early difficulties in the application of psychoanalytic approaches, the complementary effect of CBT when added to effective psychotropic medications and a culture of health provision that emphasizes short-term and problem-focused interventions.

Cognitive–behavioural therapies have evolved from a brief, discrete and highly symptom-based intervention (e.g. Chadwick and Lowe 1990) to the current emphases on longer term work, incorporating deeper level constructs such as self-concept and a focus on the therapeutic relationship (e.g. Fowler et al 1995). A growing number of empirical studies have evaluated the effectiveness of these approaches for psychosis (for reviews, see Bouchard et al 1996, Norman and Townsend 1999, Dickerson 2000), and there is now a considerable literature on the theoretical dimensions and practical applications (for reviews see Garety et al 2000a, Haddock et al 1998b).

Randomized controlled trials support the efficacy of CBT for reducing overall positive symptom levels in patients with drug-refractory symptoms (Kuipers et al 1997, 1998, Tarrier et al 1998, 1999, 2000, Pinto et al 1999, Sensky et al 2000). There is preliminary evidence that CBT may reduce the likelihood of relapse (Garety et al 2000b) and level of negative and depressive symptoms (Rector and Beck 2001, Sensky et al 2000).

The cognitive–behavioural framework for understanding psychotic symptomatology should complement, rather than replace, a biological model of psychosis. In a cognitive model, psychotic symptoms represent distortions in the formation or use of cognitive sets or schemata – that is, the structures that provide a basis for limiting, guiding and organizing information. The processes responsible for psychopathology are thought to be extreme versions of normal cognitive processes (Kingdon and Turkington, 1991, 1994, 1998). In their review of cognitive–behavioural approaches to schizophrenia, Davidson et al (1998) comment that '... while the content [of psychotic symptoms] thus represents the experiences the person has a need to make sense of, the form represents possible distortions, biases, or limitations in the ways the person has been able to make sense of these experiences' (p. 9). From a biopsychosocial perspective, the psychotic process itself may create the distorted cognitive schemata. Conversely, the psychotic process may be preceded and exacerbated by existing cognitive distortions that contribute to a vulnerability to developing psychosis.

There is a growing consensus about the components of CBT that are necessary and useful. The therapeutic stance is one of active collaboration, creating an atmosphere of acceptance, curiosity and exploration. A detailed history and assessment of the psychotic symptoms is needed to guide an individualized plan for intervention, identifying those beliefs that are most amenable to change. Interventions usually include:

- coping strategies to increase the person's sense of control of, and tolerance for, the phenomena
- 'reality test' through trying to understand the beliefs that support the phenomena, examining a range of explanations and then undertaking targeted 'experiments' to test them
- treating comorbid syndromes such as depression and anxiety (Chadwick et al 1996, Fowler et al 1995, Kingdon and Turkington 1994)

Cognitive–behavioural therapy approaches lie between the supportive work common to case management in community mental health systems and psychodynamically orientated therapies. Supportive therapy emphasizes practical and emotional assistance, whilst psychodynamic approaches emphasize the therapeutic relationship and attempt to understand the phenomena in terms of manifest and latent content (Davidson et al 1998).

Limitations of cognitive–behavioural therapies

The CBT model has much to offer in working with the psychotic experiences of a first-episode patient. However, the specific difficulties faced by patients at this early stage of the disorder are not identified or addressed through this framework alone. Therapists working closely with a person experiencing recent-onset active psychotic phenomena are often faced with intense affects such as fear, anger and despair, and may be bombarded with bizarre and fragmented thoughts. These phenomena can be pervasive and confusing and hinder consistent or useful therapeutic contact. Cognitive models tend to focus on individual phenomena – an approach that fails to appreciate the degree of disintegration in patients experiencing thought disorder, hallucinations and delusions. From a cognitive perspective it can be difficult to work with the anxieties expressed by patients in this state, such as a fear of 'falling apart', spinning out of control and being 'driven mad'. The traditional CBT framework cannot easily be applied to reintegration of the person.

The cognitive model has difficulty conveying the extreme sensitivity of patients, particularly to intrusion. Existing literature has not discussed how this may influence a directive and structured approach to therapy.

Individual therapy with patients experiencing first-episode psychosis requires the combination of available cognitive–behavioural approaches, together with access to other helpful frameworks such as psychodynamic or interpersonal understandings of psychosis. The concept of 'flexible psychotherapy' (Fenton and McGlashan 1995, Fenton 2000) which assumes the therapist's ability to 'shift gears' and use a variety of interventions and strategies is of relevance here.

Individual therapy in early psychosis

The first episode of acute psychosis usually occurs in late adolescence or early adulthood. Developmental tasks confronting the young person at this age include consolidating a sense of identity, separating from family, establishing peer connections, choosing a vocational direction and forming intimate and sexual relationships. These issues are central elements in the process of recovery and the future course of the disorder, and must be considered in comprehensive treatment. Individual therapy with a young person in the early phase of illness should facilitate these developmental tasks (Jackson et al 2001).

There are many hurdles in engaging and maintaining a young person in the early phase of psychosis. Complications arise from a potent combination of age-related factors and the profound effects of experiencing disorientating and powerful psychotic phenomena. The difficulty of providing a service that meets the needs of this group is compounded by the heterogeneity of patients. Although patients may range from adolescent to adult chronologically, many will not have achieved age-appropriate levels of psychological functioning.

Trauma associated with the psychotic episode and ensuing events is an important factor to consider when treating a young person in the early phase of the disorder. The experience of psychosis may seriously impact on the developing sense of self. This can result in a search for meaning in the experience, or attempts to fiercely protect self-esteem through denial. Such issues add complexity to notions of 'insight', and should be taken into account when attempting to engage young people.

Psychological treatment of persisting negative symptoms

The STOPP programme concentrates on the persistence of positive symptoms. Negative symptoms of psychosis should not be ignored (Rector and Beck 2001). Assessment issues with regard to negative symptoms require particular attention in first-episode psychosis (Edwards et al 1998). Many of the principles of STOPP also apply to the treatment of enduring negative symptoms. It is particularly important to keep in mind the impact of negative symptoms when progressing from one phase of treatment to the next. For example, where the client is clearly experiencing difficulty in articulating and managing emotional experiences, treatment may emphasize behavioural rather than cognitive elements and proceed slowly to more advanced phases of therapy.

Psychological approaches to persistent negative symptoms attempt to minimize the contribution of social and psychological factors to their maintenance. These factors may include attempts by patients to protect themselves from further anxiety or distress through social withdrawal, blunting of emotional responses to escape emotional pain and trauma (emotional 'anaesthesia'), mental 'switching off' or deliberate attempts to block thoughts to cope with positive symptoms. They may also include physical and emotional responses to the energy expended by the psychotic experience (e.g. weakness, emptiness) and demoralization associated with guilt, shame, stigma and fear of relapse (Watkins 1996).

Key components of psychological interventions for enduring negative symptoms include:

- adapting interview and counselling techniques to allow for slower responses and cognitive impairments (e.g. audiotapes and handouts can assist the recall of important information)
- presenting patients and families with a realistic formulation of the current situation and a framework for recovery which encourages hope and realistic optimism
- eliciting and challenging stigmatizing views of mental illness
- encouraging discussions which separate the self from the illness
- enhancing knowledge of self and different aspects of identity, while affirming positive qualities and focusing on a balanced view of personal 'failure' and 'success'
- gradually increasing exposure to anxiety-provoking or challenging situations, but in a low-stress and supportive environment
- encouraging a structure and routine for activities
- gradually encouraging increased social and emotional stimulation with realistic goals and tangible rewards
- challenging self-defeating statements and beliefs
- actively treating coexisting syndromes, such as depression and post-traumatic stress disorder (Watkins 1996, Hogg, 1996)

The STOPP programme

The STOPP programme is a short-term, one-to-one approach with a predominantly cognitive orientation. The therapy usually consists of one or two sessions per week, each lasting 30–50 minutes, for a total of 6–12 months. The four phases of therapy are:

(1) developing a collaborative working relationship
(2) exploring and coping with psychosis
(3) strengthening the capacity to relate to others
(4) finishing and moving on

Patients will vary in their capacity to progress through these phases. For some patients, forming a basic commitment to the therapeutic process and entering into the routine of attending will represent considerable emotional risk and the limit of what is possible at that time. Other patients will more readily enter into a therapeutic relationship of greater depth and progress through all the stages.

For individuals experiencing prolonged

recovery, the initial crisis associated with the onset of an acute psychotic episode has probably passed. Attempts will usually have been made to bring patients and their families into a network of support and assistance, and they will have battled through the first wave of shock, disbelief, guilt, confusion and loss. A number of interventions have probably been tried to little effect, with feelings of fatigue, frustration, hopelessness, despair and isolation becoming evident. Engaging the person in individual therapy depends on offering, and then working within, a framework which expects slower progress but a very real hope of moving forward. Engagement is a process that continues throughout therapy and influences the extent of therapeutic progress.

Engagement issues relevant to the different phases of STOPP are outlined in Chapter 3.

3

Negotiating the therapeutic process

Engagement

The aims of engagement are to:

- facilitate an atmosphere of trust between patient and therapist
- develop consensus about problems or goals
- facilitate regular contact with the patient
- establish a platform for further and more detailed assessment

Each step will help to maximize the impact of the intervention and improve the outcome of treatment.

Initial phases of therapy

Patients with early psychosis are typically young people entering a mental health service for the first time. It is particularly important to spend time in the early stages of the intervention explicitly describing what may be involved in therapy, and discussing the young person's responses to these ideas. For example:

- **Be aware of the patient's ideas about what therapy may involve.**
Do you know why you have come here to see me today? Did X explain why they thought it might be a good idea for you to see me? Do you have any ideas about it at all … any guesses?

- **Define or elaborate the aims or rationale of the therapy.**
Therapists might explain that they received information from other members of the treating team that the patient was having some difficulty in managing or coping with their persistent psychotic symptoms.
Some people take a bit longer than others to get better, and these people have sessions with me to see if there is anything we can do to help them get better.
Other patients may not be able to tolerate, or have any interest in, exploring the topic of psychosis. The therapist's decision as to whether to elaborate on explanations should be guided by patients' responses to questions about their referral, presenting concerns and expectations or hopes about therapy. A simple rationale for those patients who do not appear ready to discuss psychosis could be:
Your doctor/case manager has told me that you have been having a tough time lately. I thought we'd meet together today to start to discuss what is going on for you, and try to understand it together.

- **Anticipate and acknowledge concerns or ambivalence.**
Common concerns may include fears of being controlled by the therapist, that the therapist will initiate hospitalization or other treatment if young people are forthcoming about their beliefs and experiences, or that they will be viewed as 'mad' and their delusions dismissed as false (Chadwick et al 1996). It is advisable to make the processes of therapy transparent, and to adopt a manner that is frank and open in style.
It will take a while for you to get used to me and decide whether you want to keep working with me.

- **Minimize uncertainty and ambiguity.**
The therapist should be aware of the context in which therapy is provided. This might include paying attention to how the young person feels about the working space, establishing consistent and reliable appointment times, and meeting in a quiet and private location. Expectations about the sessions themselves may be clarified by setting a broad agenda for future sessions and explaining the collaborative nature of the patient/therapist relationship. This should include a discussion of confidentiality, including its limits. An explanation of how the Systematic Treatment of Persistent Psychosis (STOPP) programme fits into the broader

treatment context and service structure is also helpful.

- **Remain aware of the potential for psychotic symptoms to interfere with engagement.**
  Engagement may be disrupted by symptoms such as specific threats from voices, or confusion due to over-stimulation in the session. Additionally, the patient may fear that the therapist is a part of a conspiracy or may pose some other threat associated with the patient's delusional system. Flexibility within sessions can be valuable, for example, to allow for breaks or a change of topic, switch to relaxation strategies, or limit the length of the session. A sensitive approach to discussing any reluctance to disclose or engage may also help (Fowler et al 1995).

- **Actively seek a collaborative approach.**
  The patient's needs and preferences should be actively sought from the first contact, but there is also a need to balance flexibility with reliability. Being very responsive to the patient's expressed wishes can eventually undermine the therapist's capacity to work. It is important to clarify the conditions in which the patient feels safe and able to exert some control, but a stance on the minimum therapeutic contact should be maintained. This process usually proves to be an important step in developing trust, and establishing a sustainable relationship that is fair to both parties.

Case example – Dale: engagement in the initial phases of therapy

Dale, aged 24, is experiencing his first episode of psychosis. Six months after entering the mental health service he continues to experience some paranoia, auditory hallucinations and delusions of guilt. He is reluctant to discuss these phenomena in any detail. Dale has been attending sessions with his case manager and doctor regularly, and has been treated with risperidone and then olanzapine. He has seen the STOPP therapist on two occasions.

Dale: It's just too much for me to come along to these sessions. I don't think I'll be able to keep coming.
Therapist: What do you find most difficult about coming here?
Dale: It's hard having to do this twice a week. It's just all too hard.
Therapist: You are finding it difficult to come as frequently as we had first planned?
Dale: Yes.
Therapist: Would it make it easier if we started off with one session a week?
Dale: I'd just like to come every now

and then when I felt up to it, otherwise I don't think I should come at all.
Therapist: I realize there may be times when what we talk about will be particularly difficult, and that you will have 'down' days when you feel worse than others. At the same time, we need regular follow-ups to work through some of your concerns and get to know each other. I could set aside a time each week and we could be flexible in how much time we spend at each meeting depending on how you feel. Do you think you could let me know if you were too uncomfortable or not feeling well?
Dale: I guess so.

The therapist will need to explore the reasons for Dale experiencing difficulty in attending. Practical issues may need to be sorted, such as tackling public transport anxiety, providing train tickets/taxi vouchers/hospital transport etc., the option of sessions being held at Dale's home (even for alternate appointments) and the offer of reminder wake-up telephone calls.

Mid-stage of therapy

In the mid-stage of therapy, it is likely that the young person will be attending sessions regularly and will be familiar with the therapeutic process. However, the increasing intensity of exploration about life experiences and relationships may leave the individual feeling vulnerable and exposed. Keep in mind the possibility that the patient may be reluctant to discuss 'personal' issues or psychotic symptoms. He or she might present in a guarded manner or suddenly miss some sessions. Raising these issues and possible concerns in a supportive and understanding manner may assist, and also provides an opportunity to explore associated emotions.

Case example – Troubleshooting barriers to engagement in mid-therapy
Therapist: I've noticed that you seem to be having difficulties attending our appointments lately.
Patient: I guess I've got a lot happening lately.
Therapist: I imagine it must be difficult to deal with everything going on in your life as well as talk about some heavy things here.
Patient: Yeah, I feel tired after seeing you sometimes.
Therapist: Sometimes it can be difficult to share things that are very personal with someone else – it can be draining and a bit scary. Do you ever find that?
Patient: Yes. I don't want to talk about

my past at all – it makes me feel really guilty.
Therapist: So, it seems a problem that you are very reluctant to discuss your past experiences, but I've been asking a lot about them. Maybe we can work out some way to deal with this problem together?
Patient: I just don't want you to ask me too much about the bad things I've done.
Therapist: Because those bad things cause you distress?

Closing stages of therapy

The final sessions of therapy might raise specific concerns for the young person about ending the relationship and moving on, and it is vital to ensure a smooth transition. These final sessions:

- have the potential to influence the patient's ability to engage in further therapeutic contact
- provide the opportunity to consolidate learning
- reinforce techniques for, and instil a sense of competence in, managing symptoms and life events

Providing a structure in which patients are aware of planned time-lines for STOPP therapy can assist in preparing for final sessions. It is also important to discuss realistic expectations about therapeutic outcomes. For example, when only brief interventions are possible, individuals need a clear explanation about what can be achieved in a short time-frame. Some of these issues can be discussed at the outset, then reinforced later during the course of the programme.

Factors which can facilitate closure include:

- regular discussion during the course of therapy about time-lines and the expected number of sessions
- discussion in the final sessions about ongoing sources of emotional and other support
- review of progress to date and areas of mastery that have been achieved
- reflection on the sense of loss that may be associated with ending the therapeutic relationship

For further reading on engagement see:

- Chadwick P, Birchwood M, Trower P (1996) *Cognitive therapy for delusions, voices and paranoia* (pp. 37–44). Chichester: Wiley.
- EPPIC (2002b). *Cognitively-Oriented Psychotherapy for Early Psychosis: Manual 4 in a Series of Early Psychosis Manuals.* Early Psychosis Prevention and Intervention Centre: Melbourne.

- Fowler D, Garety P, Kuipers E (1995) *Cognitive behaviour therapy for psychosis: theory and practice.* Chichester: Wiley. (Especially Chapter 9.)
- Kingdon D, Turkington D (1994) *Cognitive-behavioural therapy of schizophrenia.* New York, NY: Guilford Press.
- Safran JD, Muran JC (2000) *Negotiating the therapeutic alliance: A relational treatment guide.* New York, NY: Guilford Press.

4

Phase 1: Developing a collaborative working relationship

Aims

The first phase of the Systematic Treatment of Persistent Psychosis (STOPP) therapy, which proceeds in tandem with engagement, aims to:

- establish a space for the therapy that is clear and safe
- conduct an assessment
- develop a psychological formulation about the young person's presenting concerns
- facilitate the progress of therapy to the next phase

The assessment that occurs throughout this phase should assist patients to realize that it is possible for their experiences to be understood, and that enhanced understanding might be beneficial. The psychological formulation includes initial hypotheses about factors that may have contributed to the development of the psychotic illness, the nature of the psychotic phenomena and factors that may contribute to ongoing symptoms. This formulation may be further elaborated and refined as more information is obtained during the course of therapy.

An agenda for therapy should be established, based on an agreement to work together for a stated purpose. The agenda should offer patients a way to make sense of their situation by discussing the case formulation and outlining how therapy can help. Typically, this process will generate three or four specific areas on which to work together.

Common difficulties and obstacles

Common difficulties or obstacles in developing a collaborative working relationship include:

- the individual's feelings of hopelessness, despondency and despair about recovery and treatment
- the nature of the psychotic phenomena, which may limit the development of trust
- the patient's caution or fear about discussing personal matters
- stigma issues, such as fear of appearing 'mad' or 'dumb'
- discomfort and unfamiliarity with therapy
- therapy confirming a sense that recovery is not progressing as well as hoped
- confronting a need to change
- previous experiences of pain associated with trusting others
- unpleasant or unhelpful therapeutic contacts in the past

Therapists can anticipate such concerns, making it clear that they can be talked about and offering reassurance around the intention of therapy.

Areas of focus

Areas of focus in the first phase are assessment, formulation and development of an agreed agenda for continued work.

Assessment

Clinical assessment in the initial phase of STOPP therapy should develop, from a psychological perspective, a detailed understanding of the patient's view of current difficulties, entry into treatment for mental health problems and progress to date.

Assessment instruments

Routine psychiatric assessment should have occurred well before the young person commences STOPP therapy. However, additional and specific assessment instruments can enhance the depth of information obtained and offer ways to evaluate the effects of therapy. Some instruments to consider include the following:

- General psychopathology
  - 24-item Brief Psychiatric Rating Scale (BPRS-E; Lukoff et al

1986, Overall and Gorham 1962, Overall 1988)
  - Revised Beck Depression Inventory (BDI-IA; Beck and Steer 1993) or Beck Depression Inventory-II (BDI-II; Beck et al 1996a,b, Steer et al 1997)
- Positive and negative symptoms
  - Global Scale of Delusional Severity (GSDS; John et al in preparation) which is a modification of the Maudsley Assessment for Delusions Schedule (MADS; Buchanan et al 1993)
  - Beliefs About Voices Questionnaire (BAVQ; Chadwick and Birchwood 1995)
  - Psychotic Symptom Rating Scales (PSYRATS, auditory hallucinations subscale and delusions subscale; Haddock et al 1999)
  - Scale for the Assessment of Negative Symptoms (SANS; Andreasen 1984).
- Knowledge about psychosis
  - Knowledge of Psychosis Questionnaire (Birchwood et al 1992)
- Coping skills
  - Antecedent and Coping Interview (Tarrier 1992)
  - Coping Strategies List (Farhall and Voudouris 1996, Farhall and Gehrke 1997)

Cognitive–behavioural framework

Cognitive–behavioural frameworks can be useful in mapping the features of specific psychotic symptoms, and the internal and external factors related to an occurrence or exacerbation of the phenomena. Our approach to assessment in this regard is similar to that of Fowler et al (1995).

Cognitive behavioural analysis carefully assesses the nature and quality of the problems experienced, the antecedents or triggers related to onset of symptoms and the consequences of the experience. Preliminary questions, such as "Have you ever heard noises/voices that no-one around you could hear?" can be used to commence a cognitive–behavioural assessment interview.

The assessment aims initially to identify the experiences that cause most distress to the patient and clarify these concerns. The therapist carefully explores the *frequency* and *duration* of the symptoms and the *circumstances in which such symptoms occur.* Additional questions may reveal the *features of the experience* (e.g. loudness of voices). Information about the *content of the voices, delusional beliefs or misinterpretations* is gathered in detail, together with information on the *conviction in*, and *preoccupation with*, the phenomena.

Because each patient will interpret the experience from their unique perspective, an assessment of its *meaning* to the individual is vital. The assessment of *emotional responses* to such experiences will reveal:

- the *intensity* of the experience
- the *type of emotion* evoked (sad, angry, frightened, soothed etc.)
- the *personal significance* of the experience
- the person's *reaction* to such experiences (screaming, running away etc.)

Careful exploration of the young person's *beliefs* about the psychotic experiences can help to make sense of their responses and reveal important information about how they view themselves and the world around them (Chadwick et al 1996, Fowler et al 1995, Peters et al 1999).

Some useful questions are included in the text box.

Cognitive–behavioural framework for assessment

Useful questions may include:

Frequency

"How many times does it occur during the day?"

Duration

"How long does it last?"

Circumstances in which symptoms occur

"Where were you when this happened?"

"Are you most likely to have this experience when you are alone or with others?"

Features of the experience

"Was the voice as loud as mine?"

"Could you hear it clearly, or was it muffled?"

"How convinced were you that you were being watched?"

"Can other people hear them?" If not, "Why do you think that?"

Content of the voices, delusional beliefs or misinterpretations

"Exactly what do the voices say to you?"

"Where do you think that the voices come from?"

"How did you come to the conclusion your phone was bugged?"

Emotional responses

"How did it make you feel?"

Personal significance

"Did this make you believe more strongly that there is a conspiracy against you?"

"How did this confirm that you were evil?"

Reaction to the experience
"How much time did you spend preoccupied with trying to work out the puzzle?"
"What did you do about it?"
"Did you believe you had any control over what was going on?"

Case example – Jenny: cognitive–behavioural assessment of voices

Jenny and her therapist have completed several sessions that have focused on cognitive–behavioural assessment of Jenny's experience of voices.

Together, they identified that Jenny experiences a number of very critical voices daily, which she believes are those of family members *[number of voices, frequency, content and attribution/personal significance]*. They occur several times a day and are usually moderately loud and close to her ears, although at times they scream her name – frightening her *[features of the symptoms]*. These experiences usually last for a few minutes, but can last for up to an hour *[duration]*. The voices are generally experienced when Jenny is alone and seem to occur more frequently (or be exacerbated) in the context of extreme anxiety when anticipating a task she perceives as very important *[antecedents]*. The voices typically make derogatory or critical comments such as "Can't you work it out?", "How stupid are you?", "You shouldn't have done that!", "Dumb, dumb, dumb!" *[content]*.

Jenny responds to these situations in varying ways. At times, she can laugh it off and ignore a comment. At other times, she becomes very frustrated and annoyed with herself and finds herself agreeing with the comments and feeling depressed *[consequences]*.

Experiences of trauma

For many individuals with first-episode psychosis, the experience of psychosis itself may be a traumatic event that disrupts developmental tasks and life experiences and challenges the sense of self (Jeffries 1977, Jones et al 1986). A trauma framework can be useful for recognizing the enormous impact of becoming unwell, remaining unwell and coming into treatment. During the course of assessment and intervention, it is important to be aware that the young person may have experienced, or be currently experiencing, posttraumatic stress disorder (PTSD; McGorry et al 1991). The experiences of restraint, hospitalization or sedation may have long-term impacts on the patient. Sensitivity to the signs and symptoms of PTSD and their relationship to some of the phenomena observed in early psychosis may facilitate more effective interventions.

Not surprisingly, it is common for patients experiencing a prolonged recovery to avoid thinking about the psychotic experience. During assessment, it is important to recognize a person's unwillingness to discuss these sensitive issues. At times, their denial may need to be respected. However, since emotional responses to psychotic phenomena are dynamic in nature, the therapist may use opportunities in future sessions to return to issues previously considered too distressing.

Signs that may be a consequence of PTSD include:

- the tendency to either 'integrate' ("psychosis is me") or 'seal-over' ("I never had psychosis") the psychotic experience
- avoidance of places and situations which trigger unpleasant memories
- psychic 'numbing'
- disruption to identity and sense of self
- a sense of confusion about current, past and potential identity and future, which may ultimately be detrimental to the developing personality
- difficulty in integrating perceived societal views of mental illness, which are often seen to be unsupportive or stigmatizing

In patients with PTSD, moving forward may require a search for meaning in the experience, confrontation of fears about facing the future, the development of a sense of mastery over the experience and support from significant others (Jackson et al 2001). Practical approaches to addressing these issues during treatment are outlined in Chapters 5 and 6.

Personal and family history

A review of the individual's personal and family history should develop an understanding of personality functioning, sense of identity and developmental stage. This information is important for several reasons:

- Difficulty in negotiating developmental tasks or in establishing and maintaining relationships may impede the patient's ability to manage life stressors, which can increase the complexity of treatment and help maintain psychotic symptoms.
- Poor relationship experiences may hinder engagement with the therapist.
- The person's early experiences play a key role in the formation of beliefs about the world, self and others. Early experiences can provide valuable information for later in therapy when belief modification can become an important intervention.
- Background experiences can increase individuals' vulnerability and fragility, and reduce the capacity for recovery. Factors such as a lengthy history of substance misuse, relationship difficulties and reduced capacity to cope with stressors may maintain

ongoing symptoms. In addition, the extent of psychological 'damage' experienced throughout life prior to psychosis provides valuable information for the therapist regarding the 'pace' of therapy. Many young people are delayed in their psychological growth and require adaptation of therapy to meet their developmental needs.

Special attention should be paid to any evidence of trauma and neglect in the early history, the quality and development of relationships with primary carers in early and late childhood and success (or otherwise) in negotiating the tasks of adolescence.

An assessment of current family (or caregiver) functioning is also useful in identifying how the family dynamic might affect work with the client. It will also guide how much, and in what ways, the family could be involved in providing information or in providing support after STOPP has ceased. Families are usually well intentioned (and this needs to be reinforced by feedback), although sometimes their ways of helping may require gentle modifying. Challenging family scenarios that might be encountered include:

- 'colluding' – fear of disagreeing with the young person's beliefs about the psychotic phenomena, resulting in either active or passive agreement with the patient
- 'nursing' – maintaining a stance that individuals are 'sick' and must take their medication, which sometimes sets up an active resistance in patients, who perceive themselves as struggling against a hostile world
- 'too involved' – the desire to protect may inhibit the young person exploring the world and developing independence

It should be emphasized that families generally have a willingness and ability to support the work of therapy and simply need guidance on how they can participate in facilitating recovery. Assessment of personal and family history will determine the approach the therapist and patient feel will most benefit their work together (Gleeson et al. 1999).

Possible strategies for addressing family needs may include:

- Providing 'update' sessions with the family, for example, by involving them in one of the assessment interviews, meeting half way through therapy to discuss progress and meeting again for a closure and hand-over session.
- Providing separate family therapy or education sessions about psychosis and its treatment. These family meetings could occur with a different therapist. If STOPP is conducted separately to case management, the case manager may undertake this role.
- Linking families to others with similar difficulties through a support group.

✓Check box

A successful assessment will have:

- ☐ established an understanding of the nature of psychosis for this person
- ☐ identified predisposing and precipitating factors associated with psychosis
- ☐ explored the degree of stigma experienced
- ☐ obtained a detailed account of the phenomena (e.g. patterns, features, triggers)
- ☐ clarified the young person's explanatory model for the symptoms (e.g. how things are connected, what aspects fit together and what parts are puzzling, which components seem quite fixed, and which components allow some questioning)
- ☐ assessed the severity of comorbid difficulties (depression and suicidal thoughts, anxiety, post-trauma symptoms, drug and alcohol use, aggression and homicidal thoughts)
- ☐ obtained a clearer understanding of personality features and style
- ☐ taken account of developmental phase and complexity of identity formation
- ☐ considered possible functional components of the persisting symptoms
- ☐ identified the patient's coping resources and style
- ☐ discussed the patient's beliefs about, and experience of, treatment to date
- ☐ identified family and social supports
- ☐ explored the experience of previous relationships, including therapeutic relationships

Case example – Andrew: summary of assessment information

Andrew, a 28-year-old unemployed man, was referred to STOPP therapy by his case manager because of persisting auditory hallucinations and paranoia *[nature of symptoms]*. The family history reportedly included a lot of violence. Andrew said that he was physically and sexually assaulted by his father as a child, causing disruption to early school life *[experience of previous relationships]*. He was treated as a child for aggression, hyperactivity, difficulties with peer relationships and with schoolwork. He was referred to a special school but his IQ was found to be too high for enrollment *[coping resources and style]*.

Andrew says he first heard voices at the age of 8 or 9 when his younger brother died in a car accident *[?precipitating factor]*. He describes feeling responsible at times (particularly at Christmas) for his brother's death, his parent's separation and his mother's 'beltings'. He believes his father blames him for these events and he continues to feel anger and bitterness toward his father for his childhood abuse *[coping resources and style].*

Andrew left school at 16 and has been on the disability pension since age 24 because of back pain from a car accident. He has had four failed de facto relationships, and been charged with assault for previous aggressive outbursts *[experience of previous relationships, coping resources and style, social supports, comorbid difficulties].*

Four years ago Andrew experienced a 'nervous breakdown' involving a range of psychotic symptoms *[patient explanatory model].* He describes this as a significant turning point for him. The experience coincided with his de facto leaving him and taking his children *[trigger].*

He presented at the mental health service a few months after the breakdown, with a 2-year history of paranoia and auditory hallucinations. Andrew claims that this is a conservative record of his symptoms and that his voices and paranoia had been progressively worsening in intensity over the past 3–4 years *[duration of untreated illness].*

Andrew currently lives in a half-way house but has conflict with co-residents. Symptoms worsen at night following a difficult day interacting with others and at Christmas time *[triggers, vulnerabilities to escalated symptoms].*

Formulation

The psychological formulation provides initial hypotheses about factors that may have contributed to the young person becoming psychotic, exhibiting particular psychotic phenomena and continuing to exhibit psychotic symptoms. These hypotheses are woven into a cohesive 'story' about how the person came to present in this way at this time.

The aim of the formulation is to help the young person 'make sense' of the current situation, and to establish a rationale for taking certain courses of action in therapy. Formulations can range in complexity from brief summary statements with which the patient can identify, through to complex biopsychosocial accounts that include a diagnosis, prognosis and treatment plan, such as might be contained in a psychological report. An example of a brief formulation, especially suited to someone who has yet to come to terms with a psychotic illness, is:

> *I have had many stressors in my life and I have found it hard to cope with them. When I get very stressed these days, I hear voices. I have difficulty knowing how to respond to them, and it may be helpful for me to learn more effective ways to cope.*

For the purposes of STOPP, it is important to create a collaborative formulation that helps to provide a rationale and basis for the interventions that are to follow. The formulation could be written together on a computer such that the document can be edited and retained. This is particularly important when a lack of compliance with treatment has contributed significantly to the unresolved psychotic symptoms. The formulation may be developed and revised throughout the course of therapy as the young person comes to understand their illness better or as the therapist gains an increased understanding of the circumstances related to the psychosis.

✓Check box

A useful formulation will describe:

- ☐ key or core predisposing factors for developing psychosis
- ☐ key or core precipitating factors prior to the onset of the first episode
- ☐ ongoing triggers or antecedents which exacerbate symptoms
- ☐ possible maintaining factors – why is psychosis *prolonged* in this particular young person?
- ☐ content and specific nature of psychotic symptoms
- ☐ the personal meaning of the psychotic experience and how it relates to sense of self
- ☐ existing psychological resources, strengths and coping strategies

Case example – Andrew: psychological formulation

Andrew, aged 28, has a history of experiencing and witnessing physical and sexual abuse within his family. He first heard voices at age 8 or 9 and says their onset coincided with his younger brother's accidental death 19 years ago *[predisposing factors]*. Andrew continues to harbour much pain, sadness and guilt regarding these events and it appears these thoughts are related to regular 'down' moods *[maintaining factors]*.

These experiences, together with Andrew's learning difficulties and relationship problems, have culminated in the development of firm beliefs about his lack of personal worth and a tendency to self-blame. Andrew presents with a fragile self-esteem and a frequently regressed manner of dealing with aggressive impulses *[predisposing factors]*. Consequently, Andrew's psychotic symptoms (i.e. paranoia, voices, confused thinking) are particularly prominent when under intense stress, usually involving interpersonal difficulties directly related to Andrew's view of himself *[antecedents]*.

On a day–to-day basis, Andrew is particularly vulnerable to auditory hallucinations and paranoia when he is feeling down and 'bad about myself' *[antecedents]*. These situations usually occur three or four times a week. At these times, Andrew is frequently prone to misinterpreting other's actions toward himself as demeaning or hostile, triggering painful memories from the past. Andrew's angry responses are his means of asserting power over painful interactions and tackling the inner hurt *[emotional responses]*. Loud derogatory voices reflect the content of his thoughts – "Do it!" (i.e. kill self or others), "If you don't do it you're a coward!" *[content and features of symptoms, personal significance of symptoms]*.

Andrew equates his aggressive impulses with psychosis – defining both as 'illness' – and finds them confusing and difficult to predict. His behaviour at times appears to him to be illogical and 'stupid' or 'crazy', and he oscillates between blaming himself for his illness and blaming his father to protect his self-esteem *[knowledge and understanding of illness and its relation to sense of self]*. Andrew is particularly dependent on those who validate his painful emotions; however his tendency to avoid discussion of these issues serves as a strong defence mechanism *[?maintaining factors]*.

Andrew successfully uses meditation at night to relax and decrease the intensity of the voices. He also tries to ignore them, with occasional success *[coping resources]*.

Developing an agenda

Once a psychological formulation about the presenting problems has been developed and discussed, the patient and therapist can consider the goals of treatment and how these might be achieved. The importance of each goal may need to be weighed against other goals to determine the most pressing problems. It might be useful to describe the goals both in psychological terms (e.g. reduce subjective distress associated with auditory hallucinations or increase self-esteem) and practical, realistic and measurable terms (e.g. increase Bob's ability to go to the shop).

Short-term and long-term goals need to be distinguished. Although both can be worked on at the same time, the young person and therapist need realistic expectations about what can be achieved in short-term therapy.

It is useful to write down these goals and decide on a date to review the plan and give a copy to the patient. In the tradition of more directed and structured therapies, this list is usually a combination of the patient's expressed wishes and suggestions from the therapist. For example, patients rarely state that they want to know more about psychosis, so the therapist might need to introduce this as a topic for discussion. Therapists sometimes develop additional agenda items for treatment, raising them carefully throughout therapy. For example, this can occur when a patient has a high sense of stigma or paranoia and wishes to avoid discussion of these symptoms.

Some patients attend sessions regularly but find it difficult to identify areas of concern because of passivity, denial of a 'problem' or other reasons. A useful strategy in this situation is to use psychoeducation materials in a non-threatening manner, for example, informing the young person that the service is interested in users' opinions about the value of the materials.

Case example – George: example of Phase 1 interventions

George, aged 22, was living at home with his parents and three siblings. He had always been shy, preferred solitary activities and avoided social events. He had left school at 15 to work at a timber factory where he remained until a few months before being referred to the mental health service. For the last 7 years his social contact had revolved almost exclusively around his immediate family.

During the last 18 months George had become increasingly distressed and anxious about his workplace. Initial vague feelings that he was no longer wanted had strengthened to the point of believing that his boss had organized people to follow him, watch him and document every move. He had heard people outside his bedroom window at night talking about him and saying they were going to 'get him'. He finally took leave from work and ruminated constantly about a series of incidents where he had been badly treated. George had great difficulty controlling his frustration and anger, and had become threatening at home.

Formulation

George was a young man growing up

in a family environment that supported paranoid views of the world and one that dealt with life crises by withdrawal into the family unit. He was acutely aware of his borderline intellectual functioning and often felt slow, dumb and wary of being taken advantage of. His strong obsessional characteristics made him a careful and diligent worker, though very sensitive to change and any loss of routine or sense of familiarity. In the context of the increasing developmental demands of early adulthood which he felt unable to achieve (such as learning to drive and developing friendships and relationships outside the family) and then a series of significant changes in his workplace environment, he developed persecutory psychotic phenomena. George's symptoms were maintained by the family environment, social isolation, a poorly differentiated sense of self and a lack of alternative ways to deal with his profound sense of inadequacy and not being able to cope or find a place for himself.

Agreed agenda

George agreed that his life had become more challenging even before he had problems at work. The recent difficulties further weakened his confidence and restricted his life to a considerable degree. His stress, fear, anger and hurt were having a major impact on him and his family. The idea was proposed that it may be possible to cope better with this situation. George agreed that he would like to get some of his concerns out of his head at times, sleep better, get less angry at home and be able to do the things he used to. He remained sceptical as to whether meeting with the therapist would help but agreed to give it a try.

The agenda was written as:

(1) learn to cope with worries and concerns
(2) sleep better
(3) get less angry at home
(4) do more things that I enjoy

Summary – phase 1: developing a collaborative working relationship

(1) Young people experiencing a prolonged recovery from psychosis may be:
- coming into contact with mental health services and therapy for the first time
- fearful of the implications of the illness for their life
- ambivalent about engaging in therapy

(2) A thorough *assessment* usually requires:
- a cognitive–behavioural analysis
- attention to developmental and family history
- definition of current identity formation and coping abilities
- checking for experience of comorbid disorders such as post-traumatic stress disorder.
- the use of one or more standardized assessment tools

(3) The *case formulation* provides the basis for making sense of the current situation and a rationale for action in therapy.

(4) Developing a *collaborative agenda* increases the likelihood of patients 'owning' and investing their energy in therapy.

For further reading on phase 1: developing a collaborative working relationship, see:

Fowler D, Garety P, Kuipers E (1995) *Cognitive behaviour therapy for psychosis: theory and practice.* Chichester: Wiley. (Especially Chapter 9.)

Fowler D, Garety P, Kuipers E (1998) Cognitive therapy for psychosis: Formulation, treatment, effects and service implications. *Journal of Mental Health, 7,* 123–133.

Jackson HJ (1993) The case formulation. A necessary pre-cursor both to understanding the case history and to the selection of management strategies. *The Bulletin of the Australian Psychological Society,* June, pp. 7–9.

Jackson HJ, McGorry PD, Edwards J (2001) Cognitively oriented psychotherapy for early psychosis: Theory, praxis, outcome and challenges. In: PW Corrigan & DL Penn (Eds.), *Social Cognition and Schizophrenia.* APA Press: Washington DC (Especially pp. 258–260.)

Kingdon D, Turkington D (1994) *Cognitive-behavioural therapy of schizophrenia.* New York, NY: Guilford Press (Especially Chapters 1–5).

5

Phase 2: Exploring and coping with psychosis

Aims

The aims of this phase are to explore the nature and impact of psychosis on patients and then to build on patients' confidence in communicating the subjective experience of psychosis and managing their symptoms. This is achieved by offering a context to reflect on the experience of psychosis. The therapist conveys the sense that it is safe to talk about psychosis and that the experience of psychosis is understandable, manageable and treatable. Much of this work involves identifying the young person's emotional states and increasing their skills in tolerating and dealing with intense feelings.

The content of this phase lends itself to a directive and educational stance. However, this approach must be managed in a flexible and responsive way in order to maximize the potential for collaboration and exploration.

Success in this phase sets the scene for discussion and modification of core beliefs about self, others and the world at a later stage. Indicators of success include an increased capacity to discuss symptoms with reduced distress and effective use of strategies to decrease the frequency or intensity of some psychotic phenomena.

Common difficulties and obstacles

Common difficulties and obstacles in this phase include:

- fear and anxiety about focusing on the psychotic symptoms
- poor concentration and other cognitive problems
- reluctance to be viewed as unwell
- 'investment' in the psychotic phenomena
- reluctance to consider a medical model of events and diagnoses
- personality issues, such as a hostile or suspicious style
- comorbid diagnoses, including substance misuse
- inadequate attention to the individual's perspective and experience
- the therapist prematurely challenging or reacting to defensive responses

At this early stage in therapy it is necessary to talk about the possibility of being unwell in a gentle and sensitive manner. The general approach is to deal with the realities in a matter-of-fact way:

> *Why are you coming to this treatment centre? What does your case manager/doctor say the problem is? Do you agree? What do you think the problem is?*

Psychosis needs to be couched as something others feel the person may be experiencing, so it may be worth knowing more about. A frank discussion might ensue about the usefulness and problems of diagnostic categories, the range of psychotic phenomena experienced by some people and the association between psychosis and symptoms such as sleep deprivation, trauma, substance misuse and stress.

Moving directly into this phase from phase 1 may prove difficult if a young person clearly rejects any suggestion of being unwell. If this is the case, it might be easier to explore other areas of concern, while regularly but sensitively using opportunities to 'chip away' at psychoeducation. For instance, it may be 'safer' to discuss relationship difficulties rather than the content of voices. When discussing other life issues, the therapist might note important patterns associated with symptoms, and assist people to recognize this pattern themselves:

> *I've noticed that the content of the voices you hear is similar to some of the things your mother might say and that before hearing the voices you are often quite upset about what she said. Have you noticed this?*

Discussion about such life events opens the opportunity to reflect more specifically on the emotions that occur before or during psychotic phenomena. Sometimes individuals may be able to pinpoint these themselves. At other times, especially when working with individuals who find it difficult to identify and articulate emotional experience, the therapist might need to speculate on what the young person felt at the time: "Could it be that this made you feel ..."

When patients are very resistant to the idea that they may be experiencing delusional beliefs, it might be possible to work 'within' their framework by encouraging less distressing meanings for events, rather than by directly challenging the beliefs themselves (Kuipers et al 1997).

In our experience, young people experiencing a prolonged recovery from psychosis frequently become quite passive and dependent in their relationships with other people and in their responses to the psychotic symptoms. This may result in feelings of being overwhelmed by, or absorbed in and guided by, the experience of psychosis. If this occurs, it can be difficult to confront or challenge the content of the psychotic symptoms. It can also be difficult for the patient to focus on relationships with others and the world. The patient's responses will be influenced by their beliefs about the nature of the psychotic phenomena – for example, they may be interpreted as omnipotent or guiding. If psychotic phenomena are believed to be omnipotent, then the patient may be genuinely fearful that the voices or other phenomena will seek retribution for trying to control 'them' or for daring to speak about 'them' to another person.

Patients often develop methods to distract themselves from anxiety about the psychotic phenomena and are reluctant to try new approaches. Difficulties in identifying, communicating and tolerating emotions may exacerbate this issue, especially where there is intense anger directed toward the symptoms. Conversely, patients may also experience a fear of *decreasing* the psychotic phenomena. For example, the phenomena might fill a void in patients' minds, help to explain confusing experiences or be a source of advice, support or even company and friendship.

It is important to establish and clarify if any of these concerns exist and how it will affect the therapeutic relationship. Learning to control and manage responses to psychotic phenomena requires motivation and practical exposure (including exposure to the experience of being in control and independent), as well as guidance and support through a process of change.

Another issue which can directly affect a young person's effective use of coping strategies is a desire for immediate results, which increases the potential for disappointment if a 'trial-and-error' approach to different coping strategies is required. In addition, some methods for decreasing arousal, such as progressive muscle relaxation, can provoke anxiety. Practice and rehearsal of coping strategies in the therapy session will be needed in patients with poor concentration and memory.

Case example – Fiona: barriers to the use of coping strategies

Fiona, aged 26, had persistent derogatory auditory hallucinations that lasted most of her waking day. Although using a Walkman could bring some relief, she did not use this coping strategy outside of therapy, to the frustration of her parents and the therapist.

Over time, it was discovered that Fiona believed that harm would come to her parents if she resisted the voices. She was very tearful when discussing these fears, as she was an only child and her parents were very caring. The belief that something bad might happen if she resisted the voices was gently and carefully challenged. Fiona was encouraged to be brave and take a risk. With her permission, her parents were informed of the situation and asked to provide additional support during the first evening of using the Walkman at home.

The case illustrates that exploring reasons for not trying simple coping strategies can uncover complex beliefs. Therapists must show respect and compassion for these issues.

Areas of focus

Exploring and providing knowledge about psychosis

In this phase, discussion about the 'cause' of psychosis aims to place it within the spectrum of human experiences and explore notions of underlying vulnerability and risk. The therapist must remain mindful that patients know they are unwell, but may still be frightened by this fact. Discussion should convey a strong sense that they are not alone, and that it is possible to make sense of psychosis and to recover. Provision of psychoeducation might have to occur in short 'bursts' and reflect the language that patients use to describe their experiences. For instance, how does the patient describe the experience of being unwell? Does the person say "When everything was weird" or "When I lost it"?

At this stage, sharing the experiences of peers with psychosis can be extremely valuable. The patient can be encouraged to meet other young people with similar illnesses, watch videos or read vignettes featuring others who have 'survived' similar situations. Emphasizing the individual variability in recovery is important for those who have started to develop a sense of hopelessness because their recovery has not been as rapid or complete as hoped. Comparisons with other patients who are also unwell can facilitate such discussions.

When non-compliance with medication is thought to contribute to persistent symptoms, motivational interviewing techniques can be useful (Kemp et al 1997, 1998, Miller and Rollnick 1991). Identifying troublesome side-effects of medication, lack of knowledge about medications or unwillingness to accept an 'illness' model can help pinpoint areas to address.

Comorbid anxiety and depression or the experience of negative symptoms can also be discussed within an educational framework. Patients experiencing these symptoms must cope both with distressing psychotic phenomena and debilitating mood-related symptoms. It can be useful to provide the patient with information about the signs and symptoms of these disorders, the ways in which they may affect well-being and their interaction with psychotic symptoms.

Case example – Sarah: providing a 'normalizing' rationale by discussing vulnerability and risk

Sarah, aged 17, has a diagnosis of schizophrenia and good insight. She expresses guilt about 'causing' her illness through cannabis use and a belief that she is particularly odd for being unable to cope with life circumstances, unlike her friends.

The therapist clarifies Sarah's understanding and beliefs about how her symptoms may have developed. They review the literature on vulnerability–stress models, emphasizing the multiple sources of vulnerability. Together, they expand on Sarah's observation that people have different ways of coping, may be susceptible or vulnerable to different disorders and respond to stress in different ways. The therapist draws several different sized and shaped 'buckets' on a whiteboard. These, she explains, represent the unique coping capacity of different individuals. The smaller buckets fill up more quickly than the larger buckets, suggesting a different capacity to tolerate the same amount of stress. The unique shapes of each bucket determine where the overflow occurs, representing the different responses of people's bodies and minds to overwhelming stress.

Sarah's experience of delusions is placed within a continuum of thoughts experienced by people in general – ranging from misinterpretations or misunderstandings of events through to delusional beliefs.

The therapist and Sarah discuss how she can learn to cope better with stressors in the future, so that her 'bucket' fills up less quickly, and how to minimize exposure to her unique risk factors such as cannabis.

✔Check box

In exploring and providing knowledge about psychosis, the patient may have:

- ☐ developed an increased ability to tolerate discussion about psychosis and tolerate intense emotions
- ☐ learned about the risk factors for developing psychosis
- ☐ identified factors that might make symptoms better or worse, including substance misuse
- ☐ learned about the variability in rates of recovery
- ☐ discussed the nature of depression, including symptoms, causes, treatments and effects on memory and thinking
- ☐ discussed the nature of anxiety, including symptoms, role of avoidance, effect on thinking and the body and the difficulties associated with dealing with strong affective states
- ☐ accepted the definition of the term 'psychosis' and its symptoms – a combination of altered feelings, thoughts, behaviours and perceptions
- ☐ discussed examples of altered perception (such as hearing voices), feelings (numbness), thoughts ("someone is after me") and behaviours (running naked down the street) and how they may be related
- ☐ developed a 'normalizing' approach to the experience of some symptoms (Kingdon and Turkington 1994)
- ☐ learned about types of medication and their effects
- ☐ discussed strategies to manage stress and substance misuse
- ☐ learned about types of psychoses and diagnoses

Coping with psychotic symptoms and emotions

Progress in dealing with distressing psychotic phenomena and emotional arousal can increase the therapist's credibility and the patient's commitment to the therapy. This section of the STOPP programme concentrates specifically on achieving these advances.

Assessment of current coping skills

The methods that the young person uses to help cope with psychotic phenomena, both past and present, need to be determined. The therapist adopts an inquiring approach and at the same time conveys confidence that coping can be improved. For example, it is possible to use examples of success with other patients who have managed to reduce or eradicate their symptoms. Perhaps the most important component of this phase is to really care about what the young person is experiencing. This will require a full assessment of the patient's experience using active listening, note taking and careful questioning.

In many cases the individual will not have previously explained the situation to this extent. The experience of the assessment process can improve self-esteem and firm identity, contributing to the idea of 'getting stronger'.

Patients can be encouraged to keep a journal, recording the time, place and circumstances when they experience their symptoms. This can assist in exploring coping responses (helpful and unhelpful), clarifying any patterns that may be evident and exploring the beliefs underlying some of these experiences (Haddock et al 1997). When a patient is experiencing significant negative or depressive symptoms, the therapist might need to rely on very recent events to obtain such information.

Case example – Simon: eliciting information about coping responses

Simon, aged 14, is experiencing his first episode of psychosis. He has kept a diary of the situations, thoughts and feelings when he has experienced auditory hallucinations. Although it still remains unclear to Simon, it seems to the therapist that he experiences symptoms during or after situations involving intense emotion such as anger, anxiety, guilt, humiliation or embarrassment. Simon also finds it extremely difficult to tolerate discussion about intense emotions, because of his fear that they may not be contained or a belief that anger is 'bad' and undesirable. Simon's approach to dealing with such feelings in the past has been to try to distract himself or 'fight' with the voices in an effort to get rid of them. The therapist assists Simon to make these links for himself:

Simon: I had a terrible day yesterday – the voices just kept getting worse and worse and then they started screaming in my head. I tried to stay calm and relaxed and ignore them but I just got so stressed.

Therapist: When did the voices start?

Simon: First thing in the morning and then they just got worse.

Therapist: Do you recall anything that might have been a bit stressful for you in the morning?

Simon: Not really, I just went off to school and met up with my friends, but the voices got quite bad so I went to the toilets. That didn't help me, so I started swearing at them to go away. By the time I got to home room, I was still having them and then the teacher asked me if I could do roll call all day. I told him 'no' three times because I didn't want to do it.

Therapist: Did you know that you might be rostered on for that day?

Simon: I thought that I might be in the morning before school.

Therapist: Did that worry you?

Simon: I was worried whether to say yes or no to doing it. If I said yes, what would I have to do?

Therapist: Did you think it would be hard to get up in front of everyone and take a roll call?

Simon: Yes.

Therapist: Is that something that kept bothering you when you arrived at school?

Simon: Yes, I couldn't stop thinking about it and then the voices kept calling me an idiot and making it worse.

Therapist: What happened after you said "no" to doing the roll call?

Simon: I felt really bad.

Therapist: When you say "bad", what do you mean?

Simon: I don't know.

Therapist: Disappointed in yourself?

Simon: Yes, I think so. Sort of dumb for not giving it a shot.

Therapist: When did you notice the voices were the worst?

Simon: In the periods after home room. They got louder and louder and kept calling me all sorts of names.

Therapist: Do you think that feeling a bit anxious about the whole thing, and then a bit down on yourself for not trying, may have been related to how bad the voices got?

Simon: I think it could have been.

Introducing coping strategies

In the STOPP programme, the therapist helps the patient to:

- develop ways to reduce physical tension
- distract themselves from their experience
- expose themselves to the experience

Patients are unlikely to initiate exposure themselves and this is the task that requires most time in therapy sessions. A trial-and-error approach is sometimes necessary to identify the most useful strategies for the individual.

Useful coping strategies for delusions or hallucinations

Reduction of tension:

- coping cue cards:
  - *Stay calm.*
  - *Think this through.*
  - *Am I jumping to conclusions?*
- relaxation: progressive muscle relaxation or similar strategies

Distraction methods:

- headphones for active listening to music
- ear plugs (for voices)
- reading aloud
- humming or singing out loud or to self
- exercise
- concentrating on the radio or television
- ignoring the voices
- talking to others
- sleeping
- concentrating on naming and describing objects in the room – out loud or to self

Focusing methods:

- observing and describing the voices – tone, content, gender etc. – and their meaning and relationship with thoughts and beliefs
- 'bringing on' the voices in sessions with the therapist and using strategies to minimize distress and symptoms (see case example below)
- graded exposure to feared situations, preferably with the help of the therapist

Other:

- Activity scheduling

(Farhall and Gehkre 1997, Haddock et al 1997, Jenner et al 1998, Shergill et al 1998, Watkins 1993)

Distraction

Most people with psychotic symptoms spontaneously try some form of distraction. It can be useful to focus on a limited number of strategies they are already using and refine the techniques so they are used more effectively and more systematically.

The most successful distraction techniques are those which involve meaningful information and cognitive processing and also use vibration of the vocal chords. Distraction techniques alone do not seem to increase patients' confidence about dealing with voices and can contribute to anxiety about them, so it is advisable to use some focusing strategies as well.

Exposure

A graded exposure to voices in conjunction with a calm and relaxed physiological state can be established. The aim is for the person to report particular dimensions of the voices as they occur (e.g. loudness, location, gender) while maintaining a consistently low level of arousal. In our experience, getting the person to repeat the content of the voices in the wording of their own thoughts (e.g. convert "you are an idiot" to "I am an idiot"), is effective, although this may prove confrontational.

Case example – James: learning to tolerate auditory hallucinations through exposure

James and his STOPP therapist have been meeting twice weekly for 2 months. During this time, James has been encouraged to keep a diary to record the circumstances before, during and after the occurrence of distressing auditory hallucinations, as well as his thoughts and feelings at the time.

The diary indicates some patterns of behaviour associated with hearing voices. He often experiences the hallucinations when he feels particularly anxious about a forthcoming event and then he becomes acutely anxious in response to the voices themselves.

James' anxiety appears to be associated with several beliefs: that he is powerless to stop, control or ignore the voices when they are present and that the voices themselves are intolerable and must cease immediately. This results in frantic efforts to do whatever he can to stop the voices, with increasing frustration and anger that these attempts do not have any effect. To his dismay, the voices often worsen in intensity, reinforcing his belief that there is little that seems to help.

The therapist and James discuss this pattern. They decide he will learn progressive muscle relaxation in sessions and practice this at home (in the absence of the hallucinations) to assist in overall anxiety management. James practises for several weeks and discovers that, with the guidance of the therapist, he can successfully be distracted from focusing on the voices.

The therapist explains that James might feel some initial anxiety when he tries this unassisted, but learning to manage the situation will eventually lessen his anxiety. He is encouraged not to 'fight' the voices, but acknowledge their presence and then focus on self-management and calming strategies.

In the session, James is asked to think about how he may 'bring on' the voices. This helps him recognize that there are some things he can do to control their onset and intensity. He is baffled at first, but then finds that 'negative' thoughts can effectively 'bring them on'.

James is initially frightened by the commencement of the voices, then somewhat worried and doubtful that they will not go away. The therapist encourages him to focus on remaining relaxed and to concentrate on verbally describing, in detail, the features of the smoke detector in the room, followed by the features of the clock on the wall. He is next asked to read a simple passage from a magazine out loud. Although he is still experiencing voices, he rates their intensity and loudness as low and his distress as minimal. James acknowledges that this level of hallucinations is tolerable and manageable.

People experiencing psychotic symptoms usually believe they have no control over their symptoms. These sorts of 'experiments' demonstrate that some influence over their experiences may be possible.

Case example – Simon (continued from earlier example): graded exposure to feared situations

Simon, aged 14, is at an age where cognitive approaches alone are difficult to use throughout the session. However, Simon acknowledges that anxiety is a problem, so he and the therapist devise practical tasks for them to do together to help Simon face his fears. For example:

- Simon and the therapist go to the shopping centre together and take it in turns to ask someone how to find a particular street. They plan together how they will prepare to do this, and talk about how it felt afterwards.
- Simon practises providing critical feedback to the therapist about her 'performance' in the previous task.
- Simon and the therapist play with puzzles and brain teasers which evoke frustration and manage this frustration in sessions.
- Simon is asked to think about a way in which he may 'bring on' the voices in a session. Simon works out how to 'bring on' the voices by using 'bad thoughts'.

Reality testing

'Reality testing' of beliefs about psychotic phenomena can help in exploring alternative explanations for unusual experiences. The process of constructing 'tests' of the beliefs helps to identify patients' ideas about the origins, cause and meaning of some of their experiences. At later points in therapy, this can lead to discussion about possible psychological functions of the psychotic phenomena and facilitate gradual connections between the content of voices and the patient's 'disowned' thoughts about themselves.

Case examples – guided 'experiments' to challenge beliefs about psychotic phenomena

David

David, a 26-year-old professional, recovered well from the affective symptoms of an episode of mania but still had distressing delusions of reference. Behavioural analysis was used to identify the circumstances in which he experienced these delusions and it was clear they were triggered by specific television programmes.

The patient and therapist examined videoconferencing equipment located on the therapy site. It was clear that the equipment needed to 'watch' someone was complex, large and very expensive. The following session, the therapist visited the patient at home with his family for a session around the television. They discussed when the television was purchased and whether there was any possibility of it being 'extra special'. The delusions were explained to the patient's brother, who then discussed the patient's experiences and helped support him as they watched the troublesome programmes together.

Anne

Anne, aged 23, was convinced that others could hear her thoughts and the voices she was experiencing. Anne had not considered the possibility that her belief may be incorrect and had felt anxious about being around old friends for fear they knew what was going on inside her head. She was asked if she thought it may be useful to 'test' the ideas on the therapist to see if the therapist could tell her what she had been thinking or hearing. Anne was encouraged to think as 'loudly' (inside her head) as she could, then to tell the therapist when she had finished. Anne and the therapist did this experiment several times, but the therapist was unable to identify what Anne had been thinking.

It was then decided that Anne would try out this experiment several times during the week with family members. She tested her mother and husband several times and they had been unable to hear her thoughts or the content of her voices. She reported a reduction in her conviction about this belief, and continued to undertake tests over the following weeks.

The use of pocket-size 'prompt' cards containing questions such as "Is this really true?" and "Where is the evidence for this idea?" can be useful in reminding patients to challenge the meaning of situations experienced outside therapy.

✔Check box

In discussing how to cope with psychotic symptoms and emotions, the young person will have:

- ☐ identified warning signs of worsening mental state, such as anxiety and agitation and depression, and discussed ways of coping with psychotic symptoms
- ☐ used some distraction techniques
- ☐ used some focusing or exposure techniques
- ☐ used methods to reduce physical tension
- ☐ become more specific and consistent in the application of coping strategies such as distraction
- ☐ considered alternative explanations for the experiences, and ways to 'test' the reality of beliefs

Addressing current life issues

A focus on current life issues can identify very practical strategies to foster a sense of control over life circumstances. This task makes use of methodical problem solving, cognitive challenging, specific skills training and psychoeducation.

Examples of difficulties for the young person experiencing prolonged recovery include the following:

- perceptions that the side-effects of medication are not taken seriously by the treating clinicians
- perceptions that family members are 'suffocating'
- concerns about the effect of recent events on a friendship
- worry about future career, work or study prospects

- telling a new employer or friends about the experience of psychosis and recovery
- dating
- initiating new friendships and social networks
- dealing with ongoing symptoms in social situations
- resentment toward the illness for making the young person 'different' to peers and 'ruining' their life
- fears about having children or getting married – will the 'mental illness' genes be passed on to the next generation?
- how to assertively say 'no' to substances in social situations

It can be difficult for patients to contemplate the possibility that symptoms may not completely go away, or may resurface again. Realistic discussion about this risk needs to be couched in a gentle and sensitive manner. An emphasis on the ability to continue with life tasks and goals despite symptoms and on gradual resumption of enjoyable activities can help challenge the assumption that the experience of psychosis is 'the end of the world'. Analogies with illnesses such as diabetes or asthma can be used to illustrate the 'manageability' of symptoms, even if they persist.

Case example – Louise: addressing concerns about the future

Louise, 25 years old, says she would like to get married and have children one day but is worried that her child could be born with a psychotic illness like her own. She ponders this frequently and finds it the source of many 'down' days for her, especially since she has a steady boyfriend.

The therapist acknowledges it is possible that Louise's child could be born with a genetic vulnerability to a mental illness. However, the therapist and Louise also discuss issues such as:

- the many factors involved in the aetiology and development of a psychotic illness
- the likelihood of her child developing or being born with a variety of other physical or mental disabilities
- whether it is indeed possible to predict or prevent certain life events occurring
- whether the experience of mental illness itself is unmanageable and 'the end of the world'.

Summary – phase 2: exploring and coping with psychosis

(1) The main *aims* of phase 2 are to:

- encourage discussion of the psychotic experience
- increase the capacity to manage symptoms

(2) A large component of phase 2 involves learning to identify, tolerate and control intense emotion

(3) A flexible educational and directive approach is strongly recommended

(4) Success at this point is vital to more intensive intervention later on

(5) Discussion about psychosis requires sensitivity to patients' perceptions of, and labels for, their experiences

(6) Common difficulties and obstacles:

- Patients' beliefs about psychotic phenomena may significantly reduce their willingness to try new techniques or discuss symptoms.
- Young people experiencing prolonged recovery may be passive or dependent in response to psychotic symptoms. Motivational interviewing, problem solving and practical guided exposure can assist.

(7) Exploring and providing knowledge about psychosis:

- Increased knowledge about psychosis is facilitated by approaches that emphasize it is possible to understand and manage the psychotic experience.

(8) Coping with psychotic symptoms and emotions:

- Careful exploration of current strategies that are either helpful or unhelpful will clarify what issues need to be addressed to improve coping.
- Useful coping strategies include methods for tension reduction, distraction, exposure and reality testing.

Case example – Phillip: summary of phase 2 interventions

Phillip, aged 23, lives with his parents and has one older brother. He describes himself as having a reserved temperament and having experienced some difficulty in establishing new friendships when his family relocated in his final years in primary school. He has developed a few close friendships over time. Phillip's mother describes him as being dependent on his family and uncertain about his capacity to manage age-appropriate life tasks.

Phillip performed adequately at school but lacked career direction and lost motivation for pursuing any further study. This, and disappointments in forming heterosexual relationships, has been a source of regret for Phillip. He has a tendency toward self-criticism for such 'failures'.

Phillip had a 2-year history of deteriorating function prior to his referral to EPPIC. The decline was apparently precipitated by a period of unemployment, cannabis use and disappointment with establishing a relationship. On presentation at STOPP, Phillip appeared ambivalent about discussing his experience of psychosis. He felt hopeless and helpless about his symptoms, which included auditory hallucinations, grandiose ideas, thought insertion, ideas of reference and general thought disorder and confusion.

Phillip has developed a very critical view of himself over time, which exposes him to excessive concern about other's opinions. This is a long-standing issue that is reflected in his psychotic experiences, including the content of his auditory hallucinations, and in his paranoia and other belief systems. It is possible that such a view of self, combined with regular cannabis use, may have contributed to Phillip's vulnerability to developing psychosis. Difficulty in securing a job, lack of a clear career direction, fear about others' opinions of him and disappointment in a relationship may all have added to his subjective experience of stress and a fear of being incapable or inadequate.

Phillip has tended to perceive psychosis as something that is overwhelming and uncontrollable. He has avoided thinking about psychosis because of fear and anxiety about what may happen if he talks about it or if he attempts life tasks while the symptoms remain. In addition, he has found it difficult to separate the experience of psychosis from himself and who he is.

He is in a state of limbo – afraid of the symptoms but unable to consider that he could continue with life despite the symptoms.

This hopelessness and anxiety helps perpetuate the problem and fuels Phillip's perception of his life as having 'ended' at 23 because of his experience of psychosis. His view of the past is regret about 'failures' and disappointments. If the psychotic symptoms are completely controlled, Phillip will be faced with unresolved developmental issues such as getting a girlfriend, developing a career and pursuing social and other interests.

Protecting factors and response to psychological intervention

Phillip attended 14 weekly sessions of STOPP. Four sessions focused on engagement, assessment, discussion about the case formulation and plans for further work. Ten sessions involved therapeutic interventions including:

(1) Psychoeducation regarding his concerns about other's perceptions of him having schizophrenia, guilt about having induced psychosis through cannabis use, worries about what schizophrenia may mean for his future and what the illness may mean about him as a person. This step also included efforts to normalize his experiences of psychotic symptoms.
(2) Discussion about strategies for dealing with intrusive thoughts and voices, including distraction and reality testing.
(3) Introduction of a stress–vulnerability model of psychosis, with a focus on stress management and the potential to approach tasks and activities *despite* the experience of symptoms rather than avoiding them *because* of the symptoms.
(4) Monitoring of situations in which voices were experienced. Phillip identified that these tended to occur when thinking about his future and getting a girlfriend, when reflecting on the past and when feeling anxious in group situations.
(5) Discussion of Phillip's beliefs about the voices he experiences (e.g. telepathy from other's negative opinions) including reality testing and psychoeducation.
(6) Role playing and techniques for managing symptoms in feared

situations such as making a phone call.

Phillip says he has been reassured by these sessions and is more aware of the contexts in which he experiences symptoms. He can successfully use strategies for symptoms such as hallucinations and is not so concerned about this issue now. His current priority is returning to work.

For further reading on phase 2: exploring and coping with psychosis see:

- Kingdon D, Turkington D (1994) *Cognitive-behavioural therapy of schizophrenia.* New York, NY: Guilford Press.
- 'Psychoeducation' (Module 9) in PD McGorry, J Edwards. (1997) *Early psychosis training pack.* Cheshire: Gardiner-Caldwell Communications. (Available via www.eppic.org.au)
- Fowler D, Garety P, Kuipers E (1995) *Cognitive behaviour therapy for psychosis: Theory and practice.* Chichester: John Wiley & Sons. (Especially Chapter 12.)
- Watkins J (1988) *Hearing voices: A common human experience.* Melbourne: Hill of Content.

Resources

- *Holding On to What is Real: A Video about Schizophrenia.* Available from: Marcom Projects, P.O. Box 4215, Loganholme 4129, Queensland, Australia, www.marcom.com.au
- SANE Australia (2000). *The SANE Guide to Psychosis: A guide to schizophrenia and other psychotic illness (ISBN 1 875182 47 0).* SANE Australia: Melbourne (www.sane.org).

6

Phase 3: Strengthening the capacity to relate to others

Aims

The primary aim of the third phase of STOPP therapy is to increase the patient's sense of integration. This is achieved by assisting the patient to differentiate and consolidate aspects of self and actively address the psychotic beliefs about others.

A secondary aim is to increase understanding of the process of therapy and facilitate the therapeutic encounter with the therapist, by maximizing opportunities for thinking together and self-reflection.

Common difficulties and obstacles

Common difficulties and obstacles in this phase include:

- problems in articulating experience
- intolerance of self-exploration
- restricted life experiences
- poor premorbid sense of self

Difficulties in articulating experience

This phase encourages greater degrees of personal participation and self-expression, which may prove challenging for the patient. For some, this results from limitations in putting words to experiences or a lack of experience in doing this. For others, the interference caused by positive symptoms allows limited room for identifying their sense of self. A range of strategies can be tried to overcome these difficulties – for example, beginning with more structured tasks or trying to leave more 'space' for the individual's own thoughts. Using non-verbal mediums of expression, such as drawing, can sometimes assist the process. Psychotic symptoms may increase during these sessions, and the development of coping strategies prior to or during such work may be needed.

Case example – Troy: difficulty articulating and expressing self

Troy adopted a pattern in which he allowed other family members to speak for him and was reluctant to state his own views or opinions. The pattern was established before the onset of his psychotic illness, but worsened when he became unwell. His family willingly continued their role and made little attempt to encourage Troy to speak for himself, because this appeared to increase his anxiety and exacerbate his symptoms. Troy's symptoms included persecutory ideas, extreme anxiety, ideas of reference and fears of humiliation.

In therapy sessions he frequently asked, "What do you think?" when posed with a question or when faced with a dilemma. If pressed for a comment or a commitment to a course of action, Troy would often say, "I don't know, I'll have to ask my Dad, do you want me to get him?"

By the end of therapy Troy had begun to make small decisions and plans in sessions, with fewer evasive comments. There was also a reduction in persecutory ideas. The therapist had used a number of approaches for encouraging autonomy of expression and confidence. These included discussion of the rationale for overcoming his fears about self-disclosure and expression of opinions: the fears seemed to be associated with increases in persecutory ideas and ideas of reference, and the fears had to be faced in a graduated way to reduce his anxiety.

The therapist also used lots of 'guessing' and hypothesizing about the fears and dilemmas Troy faced. He started to make some attempts at self-expression, including the expression of difference of opinion with family members. Troy reflected on whether it was possible to have agreement or approval from others on all of his opinions, ideas or choices. Throughout, the therapist communicated curiosity about Troy's thoughts and ideas, without being too intrusive or demanding.

Case example – Gina: passive style because of interference from symptoms
Gina experienced constant auditory hallucinations that were very critical of things she had done and said. Initially, the therapist had taken a reasonably directive approach to psychoeducation, coping strategies and increasing social support. Gina had remained passive and compliant but was unable to use these strategies at key times. She seemed not to 'own' the strategies and the therapist realized it was time for a 'change of gears'. This required giving back to Gina some responsibility for the therapeutic space. She was offered the opportunity to devise her own problem-solving approaches. This initially resulted in more silences and some uncertainty in sessions, but Gina gradually became more able to hold her own needs in mind, despite the critical voices, and bring her own concerns and thoughts to sessions for discussion.

Intolerance of self-exploration

For some patients, the increased intimacy and trust required for this phase is too challenging. Regular reviews of the structure of sessions and areas of discussion can help identify whether the patient feels 'safe' within the process. If the therapist remains sensitive to any reluctance to explore particular issues, then it is possible to develop a compromise in which reasonable concerns are validated, and areas to be explored later are clearly identified. Education about the value of discussing certain topics can be useful.

Case example – Daniel: reluctance to discuss personal issues
Daniel and his father made it clear to the therapist that they just wanted strategies for coping with the symptoms and distress of psychosis. They did not think it would be useful to "get into stuff" because that approach would only make Daniel worse. His father said: "Once he starts thinking for himself, all sorts of things

get out of hand." This had been a problem in the past in relation to issues of sexuality and developing independence. Daniel's father was concerned that he would become more troublesome and less compliant at home.

The therapist suspects that if Daniel becomes more independent and begins to recover, this may result in loss and loneliness both for Daniel and his father. It is too great a risk for Daniel and his father to consider.

Restricted life experiences, poor premorbid sense of self

Re-engaging patients with interests, activities and ideas they had prior to the onset of psychosis is an important part of recovery. For a significant proportion, their lives while experiencing psychosis are impoverished and provide few opportunities for pleasure. Attempts should be made to link the young person to community resources and networks, emphasizing the social components, such as attendance at group programmes (Albiston et al. 1998, EPPIC 2002c). If social anxiety is a significant factor then group work may need to be considered.

Case example – Anthony: restricted life experiences

Anthony lived in a Housing Commission house with his parents and two siblings. His father received the invalid pension for many years following a work injury and suffered from chronic pain. His mother supplemented the family income with occasional work as a cleaner. Anthony developed few friendships during his schooling and left at age 15. His main interest prior to the onset of his first psychotic episode was working alone on his car in his garage. All his social contact occurred through the family.

This phase of STOPP therapy initially explored his relationships with family members. Articulation of ideas, preferences and dislikes was strongly encouraged and any small steps toward self-reliance were consistently emphasized. The work then evolved into a behavioural and practical form to identify and pursue activities that Anthony had never tried. He became actively engaged in exploring social options based on his interest in cars.

Case example – Phillip (example continued from Chapter 5)

In moving into phase 3 of STOPP with Phillip, the therapist set the scene by talking about developmental tasks and obstacles to usual development. Phillip was encouraged to think about any anxieties, doubts or fears about his capacity to deal with life at this point and to imagine what type of support he may need. He was asked to identify small achievements that indicated his competence and independence, for example, thinking through a problem or resisting self-criticism. 'Procrastination' was relabelled in terms of an underlying fear and not simply 'laziness'. He was encouraged to acknowledge the true difficulty in achieving certain tasks, and to set realistic goals. For example:

Goal: To go to the gym for the purpose of starting to feel fit and better about myself.

Steps:

(1) Phone the local council and ask about the bus route and how to get a timetable.
(2) Phone the gym and find out about joining and how much it costs.
(3) Decide if financial assistance will be needed, and how this may be pursued.
(4) Check out a gym.
(5) Consider frequency of attendance and whether a fitness assessment and programme will be required.
(6) Consider if a personal trainer would be helpful and if there is a way this could be paid for.
(7) Ensure that I have suitable gym clothes and shoes.
(8) Pay for a membership.

Case example – Fiona (example continued from Chapter 5)

At an earlier point in therapy, Fiona's family sought a consultation about encouraging her recovery. One of her key pleasures had been driving. The family believed that it would never be possible for her to drive again due to poor concentration resulting from persistent positive symptoms. The therapist told the family it was highly likely that Fiona would be able to drive again and encouraged them to get her car ready. Fiona attended the last STOPP session driving her own car, accompanied by her proud father.

Future planning is important in instilling hope. The therapist found a concrete way to instil optimism.

Areas of focus

Identity

Phase 3 requires a reworking of the person's history, checking for information not yet obtained and incorporating the therapist's experience of the patient to make some sense of their stage in identity formation. Assessment of achievement of developmental tasks focuses on feelings of adequacy, evaluation of parental figures (distorted or otherwise), key sources of identification and sexuality.

The patient's personal history can provide indicators of personal crisis (e.g. does the person have a sense of belonging or purpose?) or other complicating issues. It is then possible to reconsider the onset of the psychosis in the context of predisposing factors and developmental challenges. A framework for persistence of symptoms can be presented in terms of these unresolved psychological aspects, as well as ongoing social and biological factors. Strengthening the sense of self is an important way to facilitate recovery and can be offered as a rationale for proceeding with therapy.

Case example – John: exploring sense of personal identity

John lived at home with his parents and three younger sisters. He spoke about feeling good being at home: he had company when he wanted it, could mostly do what he liked and felt very accepted by his family. John had moved out of home with a girlfriend about a year ago and returned a few months later when the relationship ended. He then said he could not understand why people insisted on moving out of the family home and had a fantasy about buying the family home from his parents and living there all his life. He described himself with pride as a very independent person.

John had persisting psychotic thoughts that coincidences had a deeper message and could feel a connection with a profound force that seemed to be guiding him and waiting for the right time to reveal itself. It became apparent that these symptoms intensified following discussion of increasing responsibility and independence, for example, ceasing cannabis use, returning to work and developing another sexual relationship.

The therapist gently suggested that exacerbations of symptoms might be related to anxiety about these steps. The work concentrated on John's sense of what growing up may entail. He began to describe how he viewed increased responsibility as risking loss, loneliness and a lack of freedom, and how his identity was tied to characteristics not valued in adulthood. John was able to acknowledge that he may be worried about his capacity to make things happen for himself and maintaining relationships with others.

✔Check box

Addressing identity should assist the patient to:

- ☐ make some sense of their stage of identity formation
- ☐ appreciate the experience of psychosis in the context of their wider environmental circumstances and life experiences

Exploring core beliefs

This area of focus expands on the patient's guiding views of self, others and the world, which were explored in a preliminary manner during the first phase of assessment. Here, the therapist attempts to elicit thoughts, ideas, preferences, opinions, likes and dislikes more thoroughly, and assists with the articulation of underlying assumptions. Throughout this process, the therapist seeks to identify and explore troublesome beliefs, trace their history and then challenge them through Socratic questioning and experience – for example, through exposure to activities that allow new experiences for patients.

Case example – Sam: paranoia associated with beliefs about a bad or inadequate self

Sam had been troubled by a frequent experience of paranoia in crowds and especially on trains. Further exploration identified that Sam was teased a lot at secondary school. He felt this was because of his ability to learn quickly and a sense of being 'different'. Sam believed that when he was out in public, people tended to look at him and think he was a 'freak', even though there was nothing unusual in his appearance.

Discussion revealed that Sam believed most people were not trustworthy and that the world was unfair and selfish. These assumptions resulted in his feeling very guarded around groups of people he did not know. Sam's history had been full of experiences of unfair, deceptive and rejecting behaviour from others, including his parents. He had come to wonder what this meant about him and whether he was indeed inadequate or at fault. He oscillated between being painfully hurt emotionally and lashing out in anger and revenge at those who had done him wrong. The content of Sam's voices also reflected this theme – for instance, one type was a 'drill sergeant' firing aggressive commands about defending oneself or attacking others.

Sam was encouraged to reflect on a friend's responses to others and the world – were they the same or different to his own? Why? Was it possible that some people could have good experiences with strangers? Had he ever experienced unexpectedly positive contacts with others? Had everyone he knew rejected him or let him down? The therapist and Sam also discussed his assumptions about people's appraisals of him. What would tell them he was a 'freak' if they didn't know him? Sam was encouraged to pursue his existing interest in karate and meet new people through this activity.

✔Check box

Exploring core beliefs should assist the patient to:

- ☐ develop some understanding about the role that beliefs about the self and the world may play in their life experiences

Obtaining meaning from the psychotic phenomena

This phase introduces the notion that the young person's personal struggles may be linked to the symptoms they are experiencing. Phase 2 usually involves attempts to make general, preliminary associations between emotional arousal and an increase in the intensity of the phenomena. In phase 3, the connection is elaborated by linking emotional states with particular personal struggles and the experience or intensification of psychotic symptoms.

Sometimes it is not appropriate or useful for therapists to share their psychological understanding of the psychotic symptoms with the patient, as some patients remain resistant to such concepts and communicating such an understanding may have no impact on behaviour. For example, a young person may deny any concerns about what others think about his sexual orientation, yet informs the therapist that he only told his mother of his homosexuality after his father had died. The incongruity between behaviour and stated beliefs suggests that the young man may be more concerned about this issue than he is able to admit. In such an instance it is helpful for therapists to use their hypotheses to guide interventions and take a gradual approach to building rapport and trust.

The therapist should be an active participant in the patient's search for meaning, for example, by accompanying the patient on a visit to a library to seek information or facilitating a conversation with an outside 'expert' in a particular area. This can be a concrete way to indicate that this pursuit is valuable and that the therapist is committed to making sense of an experience.

Case example – Jason: confronting fears of death

Jason, aged 26, was preoccupied with delusional guilt and persecutory ideas that others wished to kill him for things he said about them. Jason was diagnosed 7 years earlier with a life-threatening illness but treated successfully. However, 3 years prior to presentation to EPPIC, he began to experience some physical health problems and had developed the false impression that the treatment he received would continue to have a deleterious effect on his health and may eventually kill him. He presented with a 12-month history of aggressive outbursts and suspiciousness and a 3-month history of delusions. His outbursts had been in the context of extreme anger, fear and grief.

The STOPP therapist suspected that Jason's preoccupation with others wanting to kill him may have deflected some of his own uncertainty that life could end at any time. Over the course of therapy, this hypothesis was gradually and sensitively raised with Jason. He was encouraged to clarify information about his past medical treatment and current state of health with medical experts in the field. Consistently, the feedback was that the treatment would not kill him and that he was healthy.

Jason's justified anger and fear were validated by the therapist in sessions and placed within the context of understandable grief reactions. He gradually developed his own set of challenging self-statements for use when he found himself ruminating on guilt themes: "There's no use beating myself up about things I've done in the past – it only makes me feel bad and doesn't help me now."

Jason conceded toward the end of therapy that he was unlikely to die from his past illness and was less preoccupied with delusions of guilt. He was still concerned he might hurt someone again but had decided that taking his medication would help prevent this. He also maintained, to a lesser degree, the belief that someone may try to hurt him, but had decided not to be preoccupied with such concerns.

Case example – Gail: identifying a link between erotomanic fantasies and personal inadequacy

Gail had been making earnest attempts to break away from her past but had deep concerns about her goodness and capabilities. Moves to better herself invariably precipitated elaborate paranoid thinking and erotomanic fantasies which thwarted these efforts. Over time, she began to identify an increasing fear of retaliation as she made moves forward. The feelings of uncertainty about what might happen and an altered sense of herself produced much panic. This feeling then crystallized into being sure she was being followed and watched by people to see if she would 'stuff up'.

Gail found some relief in identifying who was threatening her at present. This attention also made her feel important and she fantasized about being with a successful person. Such fantasies eased her fear of being incompetent and helped her believe she would be saved and looked after.

✔Check box

- ☐ Obtaining meaning from psychotic phenomena should encourage the patient to:
- ☐ consider a link between personal struggles, emotional states and psychotic phenomena

Summary – Phase 3: strengthening the capacity to relate to others

(1) The main aims of phase 3 are to:

- increase the patient's sense of personal integration
- increase understanding of the therapy process

(2) Difficulties in *articulation of experience, intolerance of self-expression, restricted life experiences, social anxiety* and *poor premorbid sense of self* can all prove obstacles to this phase.

(3) Exploring developmental tasks related to *identity* formation can facilitate understanding of the psychotic experience within the context of personal history. Persistent symptoms may be linked to unresolved psychological and social factors.

(4) Exploration of *beliefs regarding the self, others and the world* can help

to identify unhelpful or misinformed ideas that may be reflected in the content of psychotic phenomena.

(5) Making links between personal struggles (e.g. fears, pressures) and ongoing symptoms can help to develop a *sense of meaning* in the psychotic experience.

For further reading on phase 3: strengthening the capacity to relate to others, see:

- Chadwick P, Birchwood M, Trower P (1996) *Cognitive therapy for delusions, voices and paranoia.* Wiley: Chichester, especially Chapters 4–7.
- Fowler D, Garety P, Kuipers E (1995) *Cognitive behaviour therapy for psychosis: Theory and practice.* Wiley: Chichester, especially Chapters 13 and 14.
- Roberts G (1999) The rehabilitation of rehabilitation: a narrative approach to psychosis. In: Roberts G, Holmes J, eds. *Healing stories: narrative in psychiatry and psychotherapy,* (Oxford University Press: Oxford) 152–180.

7

Phase 4: Finishing and moving on

Aims and strategy

This final phase aims to finish the STOPP relationship in a way that allows aspects of the work to be retained and kept 'alive'. The young person is re-orientated toward identifying and establishing resources that can support the progress that has been made. There is also an emphasis on cultivating detailed plans for the near and distant future.

If this phase is completed successfully, patients should be able to talk about what they have valued about the contact, identify what they take with them and express feelings about the less satisfying or desirable aspects of the process. Patients should also be able to consider what they might wish to continue working on and how. Some ideas for the future and how they may be worked towards would also have been discussed.

Finishing sessions needs to be planned well in advance. Ideally the duration of therapy should be discussed at the beginning of treatment, revisited mid-way and then focused upon towards the end of the intervention. A phase-out approach may be appropriate with the individual being able to choose the frequency of sessions in the termination phase. For example, when the therapy is near the end the young person may be given options – weekly, fortnightly or monthly contacts? Two or three meetings to complete therapy? Routine or celebratory venue for the closing session?

Patients and therapists need to be aware that continuing improvement in psychotic symptoms in the months after therapy has finished can be expected (Kuipers et al 1998, Sensky et al 2000).

Common difficulties and obstacles

Common difficulties and obstacles in this phase include:

- minimizing, or not wanting to process, the experience of finishing
- avoiding finishing (not attending)
- feeling lost, abandoned and angry in response
- increased psychotic symptoms because of the emotional distress of finishing
- limited external resources to draw upon
- therapists dealing with their own reactions (disappointment, relief, undervaluing, overvaluing)

Ending a therapeutic relationship presents issues similar to those that arise when any other relationship ends. Each patient has a unique set of previous experiences of leaving or being left behind. They will also have their own set of feelings about what the therapeutic experience has meant for them. For some, the final sessions may be too difficult to face, resulting in a series of cancelled appointments or failed attendances. For others, a sense of abandonment may evoke angry or sullen responses. Some may present with an outward bravado and be reluctant to discuss what the sessions have meant to them. Sometimes the stress of such an experience may cause a temporary increase in psychotic symptoms.

This may prove a particularly difficult phase for the young person who has experienced previous unsatisfactory closures in relationships or other significant losses. The final stages of therapy may also be a difficult time for the young person who displays dependency traits, even if these issues have been discussed and addressed in advance. The possibility of being left 'alone' to deal with life may be highly anxiety provoking. Even patients who were independent and resourceful prior to the onset of their illness may find themselves feeling inadequate in the face of what appear to be uncontrollable symptoms and be fearful of the loss of a confidante, 'coach' and support person.

Therapists may find it difficult to 'let go', for reasons such as disappointment with the progress made or anxiety about the patient's ability to manage alone. Alternatively, some may feel a sense of relief that they no longer have to see a challenging patient. Such issues require careful and sensitive attention. The effectiveness with which they are managed may affect the patient's overall experience of therapy and future therapeutic relationships.

Case example – engagement in the closing stages of therapy

Therapist: We're going to be finishing up in the next couple of sessions. Sometimes it can be really hard to say goodbye when you've talked with someone about lots of things. How do you feel about ending the sessions?

Patient: It's OK. I think I learned a bit from them.

Therapist: Do you have any questions or concerns about what might happen after we finish up?

Patient: Yeah, I'm wondering if there will be anyone I can talk to about what to do with the voices.

Therapist: Would it be helpful for us to discuss some options regarding getting access to a support person to help you with some of the work we've started?

Patient: Yes.

Therapist: Why don't we discuss some of the things to tell another person so they can continue helping you? Then we can work out who that person might be.

Patient: OK.

Therapist: Next session, let's talk about what you think is important to continue working on and who you might prefer to work with. Then we could have a less formal meeting for the session after that, somewhere nice, to celebrate what you've achieved so far. Where would you like to meet for that?

Patient: At one of the cafés down the road?

Therapist: That sounds good.

The process of closure will vary according to the structure of the clinical service and its resources. If STOPP is incorporated into the case management role, this will be a time when the therapist and client assess the agenda for continuing assistance. Questions may include: "How will the focus of sessions change?" and "Does the case manager now need to refer on to an outside agency, such as a private psychologist, for ongoing work?"

If STOPP exists as a service which is separate from care management, it is important to remind the patient that the case manager will continue to have a central supportive role. Where case managers have taken a less involved approach, they may now need to be integrated back into a new role.

Decision making at this phase focuses on what is required to facilitate continuing progress. Questions may include:

- Was STOPP sufficient to address the main issues, and is the patient recovering and progressing well? This may indicate whether ongoing intense work is warranted at this stage.
- Does the patient need longer term therapy and what may that involve? In some instances, the patient simply requires continued support to implement specific skills. In other cases, the patient may be less anxious about symptoms but faces the loss and grief associated with the realization that some symptoms will continue. The ongoing work in that instance will need to address how to make life meaningful in the face of a potentially chronic illness.
- Will the service be provided by another therapist in the organization or by the private sector?

Decisions will also need to be made about the extent to which family or caregivers are involved in the closure process and in the provision of ongoing support. Relevant questions may include:

- Should the family continue with, or commence, family therapy? If not, hand-over would focus on enlisting other supports, such as a case manager, to facilitate ongoing support.
- If the family dynamic initially caused some difficulty, how much has it changed? Can the family now facilitate ongoing care, and how may hand-over be provided to them?
- Has the family been involved throughout the process, and if so, how can they best help now? If STOPP was seen to have been beneficial, do their fears about ending STOPP need to be addressed?

Areas of focus

Dealing with loss and disappointment

Exploring previous experiences of leaving relationships can provide a good starting point for assessing the impact of ending the therapeutic relationship and how to finish the current sessions in a positive way. The closing two or three sessions also offer an opportunity to reflect on what the patient can take away. This may take the form of a review of the most memorable aspects of intervention, what did and did not work, what issues did not receive adequate attention and what was explored in detail. Such a review allows patients to express any disappointments, which can then be explored further.

Case example – Joe: discussing the end of previous relationships

Therapist: Sometimes finishing up can be a bit like saying goodbye to a friend or someone who is important to you.

Have you ever had to say goodbye to someone and not known if you would see them again?
Joe: I had to say goodbye to a case manager and a doctor and my best mate who died.
Therapist: What were the reasons for having to say goodbye to them?
Joe: I don't really know why the case manager left. The doctor was going to have a baby. My best mate died in a car accident and I didn't get to say goodbye to him. People seem to leave my life just when I'm getting to know them and feel like I can talk to them.
Therapist: Well I guess here we are going to get a chance to say goodbye properly. Let's make a plan for where and how we will spend the last session, which is three sessions away – that is, at the end of next week. For that session would you like to go over things here or perhaps go to a café for coffee?

✔Check box – key points to cover in dealing with loss and disappointment

- ☐ previous experiences of leaving/saying goodbye
- ☐ preparation for closure
- ☐ exploring the current experience of saying goodbye

Re-focus on external and social links

The closing sessions afford the opportunity for the clinician to take a more 'back-seat', supportive approach to intervention while encouraging patients to solve problems independently. This may involve a 'coaching' role in which sources of further support are identified. Discussions could involve exploring barriers to continued support (e.g. how to speak to the treating doctor about any concerns) and considering how these can be addressed. Other content areas might include means of communicating effectively with the treating team, ways of developing personal relationships, dealing with relationship and work issues, and housing and finance options.

Case example – Tammy: planning to move out of home

Tammy: I've decided since I've been seeing you to move out of home. I'm finding it hard to stay off the dope while everyone else around me uses it.
Therapist: Do you have any thoughts about where you might move?
Tammy: I'm not sure where to go. All my friends smoke too.
Therapist: Perhaps we can check out some possible places together and you could ask your case manager to help you make contact with those places when we've finished our sessions?

✔Check box – key points to cover in re-focusing on external and social links

Identify any need for stronger links with social and support networks in the following areas:

- ☐ improved communication with treating team
- ☐ housing
- ☐ work
- ☐ finance
- ☐ recreation

Planning for the future

Planning for the future involves an exploration of past and current hopes and dreams, and their implications for where the patient is 'at' today. Many patients entering STOPP therapy will have had their hopes dashed by the onset of their illness. Some will be reluctant to plan and hope for something better in the future but others will try to move on despite fears about the potential for relapse or the impact of stigma on their ability to start again. Because of the onset of the illness at a critical stage of life and perhaps previous disappointments in life, young patients may have experienced a series of failed attempts at starting a career or developing an adult identity. Fear of future failure can paralyse action and result in a state of inertia. Acknowledging these fears, as well as gently challenging the content of some of these beliefs, is an important step. A review of discussions held in phase 3 about identity and core beliefs can assist this process.

The work commenced in phase 3 about goals can also be reviewed. What would the patient like to continue to work toward after therapy has ended? Learning guitar? Recommencing a course? Developing intimate relationships? Becoming more independent? Perhaps most importantly, who may now be available to provide the support in reaching these goals?

In some cases, feedback to the family, in the patient's presence and with their permission, about the STOPP interventions and a case formulation can be a valuable tool. This provides patients with the opportunity to listen to the therapist's observations about their fears, and the therapist's beliefs about the need to take new risks and implement the strategies that have been developed. Of course, this process also familiarizes the family with any important issues that might impede future progress.

Finally, an emphasis on relapse prevention and management is also essential at this stage. The patient is encouraged to review the early signs of worsening symptoms and the benefit of complying with medication is reinforced.

Case example – Bobby: relapse prevention

Therapist: Bobby, do you recall some of the early signs of becoming really unwell that we described in other sessions?

Bobby: I think so – getting really confused thoughts and feeling like I want to be alone all the time.

Therapist: If you get that way again, what could you do to try to prevent things getting bad?

✔Check box – key points to cover in planning for the future

- ☐ exploring past and current dreams
- ☐ looking at the disappointments associated with hopes
- ☐ identifying new fears of the unknown
- ☐ identifying supports for working toward future goals
- ☐ relapse prevention

Handing over to other team members

A hand-over session between the continuing treatment team, the STOPP therapist and the young person assists a smooth transition, transfer of information and consolidation of important areas covered in therapy. At EPPIC, a written psychological formulation of the patient's situation is compiled and inserted in the file as a formal means of summarizing the STOPP intervention. The report includes:

- a brief summary of the purpose of STOPP and context in which it was offered
- background history (including initial symptoms at commencement of STOPP)
- a summary and aetiological formulation used as the basis for psychological intervention
- a list of protective factors or strengths
- speculated prognosis
- the individual's response to the intervention
- recommendations for further input

An example of a STOPP discharge report is contained in Appendix II.

It can also be useful to explore with the patient the main areas of discussion that they recall and that meant the most to them. Patients sometimes find this a difficult task but their spontaneous answers can provide a good understanding of what was most relevant or interesting. This may not always be what the therapist expected. Where the memory is vague about important areas of discussion, the therapist can remind the young person of the key points.

Transition to other sources of care can be easier if the patient is present during the hand-over. Patients can then explain and discuss their experience of therapy with other members of the treating team.

Case example – Mark: reviewing interventions to date

Therapist: We have talked about a lot in our sessions together. When you think back, are there any things that you recall that particularly struck you, or you thought were useful?

Mark: I liked it when we did those experiments together.

Therapist: What did you find helpful about that?

Mark: It made me think maybe other people couldn't hear what I was thinking.

Therapist: What about things that didn't seem so helpful.

Mark: Using the earplugs just seemed to make the voices more muffled and me more frustrated that I was hearing those sounds and couldn't understand them.

✔Check box – key points to cover in handing over to other team members

- ☐ verbal/written hand-over to treating team
- ☐ discuss with the young person how to explain to other members of the treating team the issues which were covered in STOPP

Summary – phase 4: finishing and moving on

(1) The main aims of phase 4 are to:

- offer a positive experience of finishing a relationship
- identify and establish resources to support the person in their gains and progress
- develop ongoing intervention plans for the near and distant future

(2) The closing sessions offer the opportunity to review aspects of the intervention, discuss *disappointments* and positive experiences and process feelings of *loss* associated with saying goodbye. Summarizing sessions can also help in forming a coherent 'story' about the

discussions and how they relate to the patient's life and experiences.

(3) In these sessions, the clinician takes a more 'back-seat', supportive and coaching role in assisting *active seeking of ongoing support.*

(4) The final sessions offer the opportunity to discuss *fears related to, and goals for, the future* and consider *relapse prevention* strategies.

(5) A *hand-over* to other treating team members through either verbal and/or written feedback can facilitate the transfer of valuable information.

References

Albiston DJ, Francey SM, Harrigan SM (1998) Group programmes for recovery from early psychosis. *Br J Psychiatry* **172**(Suppl 33):117–121.

American Psychiatric Association (1994) *Diagnostic and Statistical Manual of Mental Disorders*, 4th edn (American Psychiatric Association: Washington DC).

Andreasen NC (1984) *The Scale for the Assessment of Negative Symptoms (SANS)* (University of Iowa: Iowa City).

Beck AT, Steer RA (1993) *Manual for the Beck Depression Inventory* (Psychological Corporation: San Antonio, TX).

Beck AT, Steer RA, Brown GK (1996a) *Manual for the Beck Depression Inventory-II* (Psychological Corporation: San Antonio, TX).

Beck AT, Steer RA, Ball R, Ranieri WF (1996b) Comparison of Beck Depression Inventories-IA and -II in psychiatric outpatients. *J Pers Assess* **67**:588–597.

Birchwood M, Smith J, Cochrane R (1992) Specific and non-specific effects of educational intervention for families living with schizophrenia. A comparison of three methods. *Br J Psychiatry* **160**:806–814.

Bouchard S, Vallieries A, Roy M, Maziade M (1996) Cognitive restructuring in the treatment of psychotic symptoms in schizophrenia: a critical analysis. *Behav Ther* **27**:257–277.

Buchanan A, Reed A, Wessely S et al (1993) Acting on delusions (2): the phenomenological correlates of acting on delusions. *Br J Psychiatry* **163**:77–81.

Chadwick PDJ, Birchwood MJ (1995) The omnipotence of voices: a cognitive approach to auditory hallucinations. *Br J Psychiatry* **165**: 190–201.

Chadwick PDJ, Lowe CF (1990) Measurement and modification of delusional beliefs. *J Consult Clin Psychol* **58**:225–232.

Chadwick P, Birchwood M, Trower P (1996) *Cognitive Therapy for Delusions, Voice and Paranoia* (Wiley: Chichester).

Crow TJ, MacMillan JF, Johnson AL, Johnson EC (1986) A randomised controlled trial of prophylactic neuroleptic treatment. *Br J Psychiatry* **148**:120–127.

Davidson L, Lambert S, McGlashan TH (1998) Psychotherapeutic and cognitive–behavioural treatments for schizophrenia: developing a disorder-specific form of psychotherapy for persons with psychosis. In: Perris C, McGorry PD, eds, *Cognitive Psychotherapy of Psychotic and Personality Disorders: Handbook of Theory and Practice* (Wiley: Chichester) 1–20.

Dickerson FB (2000) Cognitive behavioural psychotherapy for schizophrenia: a review of recent empirical studies. *Schizophr Res* **43**:71–90.

Edwards J, McGorry PD (1998) Early intervention in psychotic disorders: A critical step in the prevention of psychological morbidity. In: Perris C, McGorry PD, eds, *Cognitive Psychotherapy of Psychotic and Personality Disorders: Handbook of Theory and Practice* (Wiley: Chichester) 167–195.

Edwards J, McGorry PD (2002) *Implementing Early Intervention in Psychosis: A Guide to Establishing Early Psychosis Services* (Dunitz: London).

Edwards J, Maude D, McGorry PD et al (1998) Prolonged recovery in first episode psychosis. *Br J Psychiatry* **172**(Suppl 33):107–116.

Edwards J, McGorry PD, Waddell F, Harrigan S (1999) Enduring negative symptoms in first episode psychosis: comparison of 6 methods using follow-up data. *Schizophr Res* **40**:147–158.

Edwards J, Hinton M, Elkins K, Athanasopoulos O (2002a) Cannabis and early psychosis. In: Graham H, Mueser K, Birchwood M, Copello A, eds, *Substance Misuse in Psychosis: Approaches to Treatment and Service Delivery* (Wiley: Chichester). In press.

Edwards J, Maude D, Herrmann-Doig T et al (2002b) A service response to prolonged recovery in early psychosis. *Psychiatry Serv.* **50**:1067–1069.

Edwards J, Harris M, Herman A (in press) The Early Psychosis Prevention and Intervention Centre. In: Ogura C, ed, *Recent Advances in Early Intervention and Prevention in Psychiatric Disorders,* (Seiwa Shoten Publishers Tokyo: Tokyo).

EPPIC (2001) *Case Management in Early Psychosis: A Handbook* (Early Psychosis Prevention and Intervention Centre: Melbourne).

EPPIC (2002a) *Cannabis and Psychosis: An Early Psychosis Treatment Manual and Video* (Early Psychosis Prevention and Intervention Centre: Melbourne).

EPPIC (2002b) *Cognitively-Oriented Psychotherapy for Early Psychosis* (Early Psychosis Prevention and Intervention Centre: Melbourne) (Manual 4 in a series of early psychosis manuals).

EPPIC (2002c) *Prolonged Recovery in Early Psychosis: A Treatment Manual and Video* (Early Psychosis Prevention and Intervention Centre: Melbourne).

Farhall J, Gehrke M (1997) Coping with hallucinations: exploring stress and coping frameworks. *Br J Clin Psychol* **36**:259–261.

Farhall J, Voudouris N (1996) Persistent auditory hallucinations: prospects for non medication interventions in a hospital population. *Behav Change* **13**:112–123.

Fenton WS (2000) Evolving perspectives on individual psychotherapy for schizophrenia. *Schizophr Bull* **26**:137–139.

Fenton WS, McGlashan TH (1995) Schizophrenia: individual psychotherapy. In: Kaplan HI, Saddock BJ, eds, *Comprehensive Textbook of Psychiatry* (Williams and Wilkins: Baltimore, MD) Vol 6, 1007–1018.

Fowler D, Garety P, Kuipers E (1995) *Cognitive Behaviour Therapy for Psychosis: Theory and Practice* (Wiley: Chichester).

Fowler D, Garety P, Kuipers E (1998) Cognitive therapy for psychosis: formulation treatment effects and service implications. *J Ment Health* 7:123–133.

Garety P, Kuipers L, Fowler D et al (1994) Cognitive behavioural therapy for drug resistant psychosis. *Br J Med Psychol* **67**:259–271.

Garety P, Fowler D, Kuipers E et al (1997) London–East Anglia randomised controlled trial of cognitive–behavioural therapy for psychosis II: predictors of outcome. *Br J Med Psychol* **171**:420–426.

Garety PA, Fowler D, Kuipers E (2000a) Cognitive–behavioural therapy for people with psychosis. In: Martindale B, Bateman A, Crowe M, Margison F, eds, *Psychosis: Psychological Approaches and their Effectiveness* (Gaskell/Royal College of Psychiatrists: London) 30–49.

Garety PA, Fowler D, Kuipers E (2000b) Cognitive–behavioral therapy for medication-resistant symptoms. *Schizophr Bull* **26**:73–86.

Gleeson J, Jackson HJ, Stavely H, Burnett P (1999) Family intervention in early psychosis. In: McGorry PD, Jackson HJ, eds, *Recognition and Management of Early Psychosis: A Preventive Approach* (Cambridge University Press: New York) 376–406.

Graham H, Mueser K, Birchwood M, Copello A, eds (2002) *Substance Misuse in Psychosis: Approaches to Treatment and Service Delivery* (Wiley: Chichester).

Haddock G, Bentall R, Slade P (1997) Psychological treatment of auditory hallucinations: focusing or distraction? In: Haddock G, Slade P, eds, *Cognitive Behavioural Interventions with Psychotic Disorders* (Routledge: London) 45–70.

Haddock G, Slade PD, Bentall RP et al (1998a) A comparison of the long-term effectiveness of distraction and focusing in the treatment of auditory hallucinations. *Br J Med Psychol* **71**: 339–49.

Haddock G, Tarrier N, Spaulding W et al (1998b) Individual cognitive–behaviour therapy in the treatment of hallucinations and delusions: a review. *Clin Psychol Rev* **18**:821–838.

Haddock G, McCarron J, Tarrier N, Faragher EB (1999) Scales to measure dimensions of hallucinations and delusions: the psychotic symptom rating scales (PSYRATS). *Psychol Med* **19**:879–889.

Hogg L (1996) Psychological treatments for negative symptoms. In: Haddock G, Slade PD, eds, *Cognitive–Behavioural Interventions with Psychotic Disorders* (Routledge: London). 151–167.

Jackson HJ (1993) The case formulation. A necessary precursor both to understanding the case history and to the selection of management strategies. *Bull Austral Psychol Soc* June 7–9.

Jackson HJ, Edwards J, McGorry PD, Hulbert C (1999) Recovery from psychosis: psychological interventions. In: McGorry PD, Jackson HJ, eds, *Recognition and Management of Early Psychosis: A Preventive Approach* (Cambridge University Press: Cambridge, UK) 265–307.

Jackson C, Fowler DR, Birchwood MJ (2000) *Early Interventions in Psychosis: A Guide to Concepts Evidence and Interventions* (Wiley: Chichester).

Jackson HJ, McGorry PD, Edwards J (2001) Cognitively oriented psychotherapy for early psychosis: Theory praxis outcome and challenges. In: Corrigan PW, Penn DL, eds, *Social Cognition and Schizophrenia* (APA Press: Washington DC) 249–284.

Jeffries JJ (1977) The trauma of being psychotic: a neglected element in the management of chronic schizophrenia. *Can J Psychiatry* **22**:199–206.

Jenner JA, van de Willige G, Wiersma D (1998) Effectiveness of cognitive therapy with coping training for persistent auditory hallucinations: a retrospective study of attenders of a psychiatric out-patient department. *Acta Psychiatry Scand* **98**:384–389.

Jones EE, Wynne MF, Watson DD (1986) Client perception of treatment in crisis intervention and longer term psychotherapies. *Psychotherapy* **23**:120–132.

Kemp R, Hayward P, David A (1997) *Compliance Therapy Manual* (Gardiner-Caldwell Communications: Cheshire).

Kemp R, Kirov G, Everitt B et al (1998) Randomised controlled trial of compliance therapy: 18-month follow-up. *Br J Psychiatry* **172**:413–419.

Kingdon D, Turkington D (1991) The use of cognitive behaviour therapy with a normalizing rationale in schizophrenia: preliminary report. *J Nerv Ment Dis* **179**:207–211.

Kingdon D, Turkington D (1994) *Cognitive–Behavioural Therapy of Schizophrenia* (Guilford Press: New York).

Kingdon D, Turkington D (1998) Cognitive behaviour therapy of schizophrenia. In: Wykes T, Tarrier N, Lewis S, eds, *Outcome and Innovation in Psychological Treatment of Schizophrenia* (Wiley: Chichester) 59–79.

Kuipers E, Garety P, Fowler D et al (1997) London–East Anglia randomised controlled trial of cognitive–behavioural therapy for psychosis I: effects of the treatment phase. *Br J Psychiatry* **171**:319–327.

Kuipers E, Fowler D, Garety PA et al (1998) The London–East-Anglia randomised controlled trial of cognitive–behavior therapy for psychosis III: follow-up and economic evaluation at 18 months. *Br J Psychiatry* **173**:61–68.

Lewis S, Tarrier N, Haddock G et al (2001) A randomised controlled trial of cognitive behaviour therapy in early schizophrenia. *Schizophr Res* **49**(Suppl):263–264.

Loebel AD, Lieberman JA, Alvir JM et al (1992) Duration of psychosis and outcome in first-episode schizophrenia. *Am J Psychiatry* **149**:1183–1188.

Lukoff D, Neuchterlein KH, Ventura J (1986) Manual for the Expanded Brief Psychiatric Rating Scale. *Psychiat Bull* **12**:594–602.

Martindale B, Bateman A, Crowe M, Margison F, eds (2000) *Psychosis: Psychological Approaches and their Effectiveness* (Gaskell: London).

Miller WR, Rollnick S (1991) *Motivational Interviewing: Preparing People to Change Addictive Behavior* (Guilford Press: New York).

McGlashan T, ed (1996) Issue theme: early detection and intervention in schizophrenia. *Schizophr Bull* **22**:197–352.

McGorry P, ed (1998) Verging on reality. *Br J Psychiatry* **172**(Suppl 33):1–136.

McGorry PD, Edwards J (1997) *Early Psychosis Training Pack* (Gardiner–Caldwell Communications: Cheshire) (available on EPPIC website: www.eppic.org.au).

McGorry PD, Chanen A, McCarthy E et al (1991) Posttraumatic stress disorder following recent-onset psychosis: an unrecognized postpyschotic syndrome. *J Nerv Ment Dis* **179**:253–258.

McGorry PD, Edwards J, Mihalopoulos C et al (1996) EPPIC: an evolving system of early detection and optimal management. *Schizophr Bull* **22**:305–326.

Norman RMG, Malla AK (2001) Duration of untreated psychosis: a critical examination of the concept and its importance. *Psychol Med* **31**: 381–400.

Norman R, Townsend LA (1999) Cognitive–behavioural therapy for psychosis: a status report. *Can J Psychiatry* **44**:245–252.

Overall JE (1988) The Brief Psychiatric Rating Scale (BPRS): recent developments in ascertainment and scaling. *Psychopharmacol Bull* **24**:97–99.

Overall JE, Gorham DR (1962) The Brief Psychiatric Rating Scale. *Psychol Rep* **10**:799–812.

Perris C, McGorry PD (1998) *Cognitive Psychotherapy of Psychotic and Personality Disorders: Handbook of Theory and Practice* (Wiley: Chichester).

Peters ER, Joseph SA, Garety PA (1999) Measurement of delusional ideation in a normal population: introducing the PDI (Peters et al Delusions Inventory). *Schizophr Bull* **25**:553–576.

Phillips KA (1996) *The Broken Mirror: Understanding and Treating Body Dysmorphic Disorder* (Oxford University Press: New York).

Pinto AL, La Pia S, Mennella R et al (1999) Cognitive–behavioral therapy and clozapine for clients with treatment-refractory schizophrenia. *Psychiatr Serv* **50**:901–904.

Rabiner CJ, Wegner JT, Kane JM (1986) Outcome study of first-episode psychosis I: relapse rates after 1 year. *Am J Psychiatry* **143**:1155–1158.

Rector NA, Beck AT (2001) Cognitive behavioral therapy for schizophrenia: an empirical review. *J Nerv Ment Dis* **189**:278–287.

Roberts G (1999) The rehabilitation of rehabilitation: a narrative approach to psychosis. In: Roberts G, Holmes J, eds, *Healing Stories: Narrative in Psychiatry and Psychotherapy* (Oxford University Press: Oxford) 152–80.

Safran JD, Muran JC (2000) *Negotiating the Therapeutic Alliance: A Relational Treatment Guide* (Guilford Press: New York).

SANE Australia (2000) *The SANE Guide to Psychosis: A Guide to Schizophrenia and Other Psychotic Illnesses* (SANE Australia: Melbourne) (www.sane.org).

Sensky T, Turkington D, Kingdon D et al (2000) A randomised-controlled trial of cognitive–behavioural therapy for persistent symptoms in schizophrenia resistant to medication. *Arch Gen Psychiatry* **57**:165–172.

Shergill SS Murray RM, McGuire PK (1998) Auditory hallucinations: a review of psychological treatments. *Schizophr Res* **32**:137–150.

Steer RA, Ball R, Ranieri WF, Beck AT (1997) Further evidence for the construct validity of the Beck Depression Inventory-II with psychiatric outpatients. *Psychol Rep* **80**:443–446.

Tarrier N (1992) Management and modification of residual psychotic symptoms. In: Birchwood MJ, Tarrier N, eds, *Innovations in the Psychological Management of Schizophrenia: Assessment Treatment and Services* (Wiley: Chichester) 147–169.

Tarrier N, Beckett R, Harwood S et al (1993a) A trial of two cognitive–behavioural methods of treating drug-resistant psychotic symptoms in schizophrenic patients: I Outcome. *Br J Psychiatry* **162**:524–532.

Tarrier N, Sharpe L, Beckett R et al (1993b) A trial of two cognitive–behavioural methods of treating drug resistant residual psychotic symptoms in schizophrenic patients. II Treatment-specific changes in coping and problem-solving. *Soc Psychiat Psychiat Epidemiol* **28**:5–10.

Tarrier N, Yusupoff L, Kinney C et al (1998) Randomized controlled trial of intensive cognitive behaviour therapy for patients with chronic schizophrenia. *BMJ* **317**:303–307.

Tarrier N, Withkowski A, Kinney C et al (1999) Durability of the effects of cognitive–behavioural therapy in the treatment of chronic schizophrenia. *Br J Psychiatry* **174**:500–504.

Tarrier N, Kinney C, McCarthy E et al (2000) Two-year follow-up of cognitive–behavioral therapy and supportive counseling in the treatment of persistent symptoms in chronic schizophrenia. *J Consult Clin Psychol* **68**:917–922.

Turkington D, Kingdon D (2000) Cognitive–behavioural techniques for general psychiatrists in the management of patients with psychosis. *Br J Psychiatry* **177**:101–106.

Watkins J (1988) *Hearing Voices: A Common Human Experience* (Hill of Content: Melbourne).

Watkins J (1993) *Hearing Voices: A Self Help Guide and Reference Book* (Richmond Fellowship of Victoria: Melbourne) (www.rfv.org.au).

Watkins J (1996) *Living with Schizophrenia: An Holistic Approach to Understanding Preventing and Recovering from Negative Symptoms* (Hill of Content: Melbourne).

Wyatt RJ (1991) Neuroleptics and the natural course of schizophrenia. *Schizophr Bull* **17**:325–351.

Wyatt RJ, Fawcett R, Kirch DG (1989) A possible animal model of defect state schizophrenia. In: Schulz SC, Tamminga CA, eds, *Schizophrenia: Scientific Progress* (Oxford University Press: New York) 184–189.

Appendix I

A Service Response to Prolonged Recovery in Early Psychosis*

Jane Edwards MA, PhD, Dana Maude MPsych, Tanya Herrmann-Doig MPsych, Lisa Wong Grad Dip Ed Psych, John Cocks MBBS, FRANZCP, Peter Burnett MBBS, FRANZCP, Chad Bennett MBBS, FRANZCP, Darryl Wade MA, and Patrick McGorry MBBS, PhD, FRANZCP

The Treatment Resistance Early Assessment Team (TREAT) is a consultation team that provides technical assistance to clinicians at the Early Psychosis Prevention and Intervention Centre (EPPIC) – an integrated clinical research setting that adheres to a scientist practitioner model with a strong emphasis on professional development via supervision and training.[1–2] TREAT comprises senior EPPIC clinicians with expertise and interest in biological, psychological and social aspects of positive and negative symptoms that persist after an initial psychotic episode. There is an attempt to maintain a pool of six clinician consultants and departing staff are rapidly

---

*This article first appeared in Psychiatric Services 2002; 53:1067–69. Reproduced with permission of the American Psychiatric Association.

replaced. Consultation has been provided to other mental health services, including child and adolescent programs. A manual detailing the TREAT approach is available.[3]

Detection of prolonged recovery

After EPPIC clients with a first psychotic episode have been registered for nine weeks, their case manager and psychiatrist receive a written query by the TREAT coordinator to determine whether positive or negative symptoms have persisted. This method appears to reliably detect those with persisting positive symptoms, as indicated by the high concordance (97%) between case managers using a prompt sheet and an independent rater (n = 30) using a score of 4 or above on either the suspiciousness, unusual thought content, conceptual disorganization, or hallucinations subscales of the expanded version of the Brief Psychiatric Rating Scale (BPRS;[4]). If symptoms have not resolved by 12 weeks, the case manager and psychiatrist discuss the individual's treatment and progress at the next weekly TREAT meeting. TREAT also receives referrals of patients whose illness is ongoing at any time during their 18-month episode of care at EPPIC.

TREAT screened 1388 persons with first episode psychosis between July 1996 and Decemeber 2001 – that is, most of the new patients referred to EPPIC during this period. 9 weeks after entry into treatment, 561 (40%) had positive symptoms; by 12 weeks 283 (20%) did. The mean $\pm$SD age of those with positive symptoms at 12 weeks was 21.3 ± 3.7 years and 67% were male. Demographic characteristics were similar to the total EPPIC cohort. Analysis of the data on a yearly basis indicates a relatively stable pattern.

Consultation and interventions

At the TREAT meeting, the case manager and the psychiatrist inform the team about the patient's situation; the focus is on the assessment, including physical investigations, and the nature and effectiveness of interventions to date. The TREAT team then reviews pharmacological, psychological, and social interventions. Pharmacological considerations include a detailed review of medication type and dosages, and features of the response. The patient's perception of medications and compliance are discussed, along with complications such as side effects and facilitating factors such as family support of treatment. Treatment principles include four components: active pursuit of effective treatment using relatively low dosages but with the readiness to increase the dose modestly or change the drug if response is delayed beyond 6 weeks; an expectation of at least two adequate drug trials (equivalent to 10 mg of haloperidol, with a lower ceiling if side effects occur) within a 3-month period;

use of atypical agents such as risperidone and olanzapine as 'first line' treatment; and the early introduction of clozapine.

Psychosocial interventions include case management tasks appropriate to the phase of illness, psychoeducation, and psychological interventions aimed at promoting recovery and reducing secondary morbidity. The psychological considerations include the nature of the therapeutic relationship, the individual's explanatory model, and identification of underlying vulnerabilities and strengths.[5]

Recommendations may involve areas for further assessment and use of specialized individual therapy. For example, we have developed a cognitively oriented approach to enduring positive symptoms in early psychosis called Systematic Treatment of Persisting Psychosis (STOPP;[6]). It draws on the range of approaches described in the cognitive-behavioral literature, and also addresses psychological issues prominent in a young person recently diagnosed with a mental illness. Key features include youth-sensitive engagement strategies; attention to developmental tasks involving the consolidation of identity, the process of separation from parents, educational and vocational goals, and the construction of a peer group, and treating co-morbid substance misuse.

Social considerations include the impact on the family and their view of the illness, the response of the person's broader social network, and social and occupational role functioning. Interventions may include increasing access to group programs, further assessment of family stress and burden, the introduction of individual family treatment or a multi-family support group, and assistance with finding suitable accommodation if the parental home is not available.

Components of family support include exploring the impact of the psychotic episode and the delayed recovery on the family system, and on each individual member. Past and ongoing trauma, experiences of loss, and changes in key relationships are explored. The family is helped to understand their role in the treatment and recovery process, and where appropriate, to address family issues which may pre-date the onset of the psychosis. The TREAT family group incorporates psychoeducation and strategies aimed at establishing a low expressed emotion environment and improving communication and problem-solving skills.

Treatment recommendations are recorded and, as of January 1999, a clinical rating of functioning as assessed by the Health of the Nation Outcome Scale (HoNOS;[7]) is entered onto the TREAT database. A follow-up TREAT review to evaluate the effectiveness of interventions is scheduled where appropriate. If symptoms continue to persist longer-term planning is commenced.

Evaluation of TREAT

Data from the BPRS, Scale for the Assessment of Negative Symptoms (SANS;[8]) and Quality of Life Scale (QLS;[9]) were available for 98 participants. These subjects were recruited from August 1996 over a 12-month period, and assessed at four time-points after their entry to EPPIC; 81 individuals had been assessed at stabilization (mean = 12.6 weeks) and about 12 months later, and 26 of these were TREAT clients. The TREAT group performed more poorly than the non-TREAT group at both time points on each of the measures. A repeated-measures analysis of variance showed that both groups improved significantly over time on the BPRS ($F = 5.8$, $df = 1,79$, $p = 0.018$), SANS ($F = 5.3$, $df = 1,79$, $p = 0.024$) and QLS ($F = 11.3$, $df = 1,79$, $p = 0.001$), but without a significant group by time interaction, indicating that there was no differential pattern of change over time between the groups.

HoNOS data collected at initial TREAT assessment and again 3-4 months later (mean = 15.4 weeks) was available for a second sample of TREAT patients ($n = 48$). Scores on total scales (10- and 12-item versions) and the behavioral, symptoms, and social sub-scales significantly decreased between the two time points. We are implementing a routine outcome assessment system that will enable case managers to readily monitor client progress at multiple time-points over 18 months.

Case vignettes

Fiona, a 26-year-old woman who had persistent, derogatory auditory hallucinations throughout most of her waking day, did not implement coping strategies outside of therapy. Although listening to music on her Walkman brought some relief, she did not use this strategy, even when she was very distressed. Over time it emerged that Fiona believed that if she resisted the voices, harm would come to her parents. This belief was gently and carefully challenged. Fiona was encouraged to be brave and take a risk. With her permission Fiona's parents were informed of the situation and asked to provide additional support during her first evening of trying the Walkman at home. At another point in the therapy Fiona's parents were consulted about ideas for encouraging her recovery. One of her key pleasures had been driving. Her parents believed that she would never be able to drive again because of the poor concentration she had as a result of her positive symptoms. The therapist told the family that it was very likely that Fiona would drive again and encouraged them to get her car repaired. Fiona attended the last STOPP session driving her own car accompanied by her proud father.

Maria was a 28-year-old married woman who held a delusional belief that she smelled bad as a result of an infestation. She believed that people avoided her because of this smell and she was reluctant to engage in a number of previously enjoyed social activities. It was suggested that she ask three trusted people to write down three adjectives to describe how Maria smelled to them. She agreed to give it a try. All three individuals gave interesting responses – "fresh" (husband), "sexy" (sister) and "like roses" (case manager) – that left Maria surprised and a little skeptical. On hot days the therapist made a point of sitting close to Maria, telling her that she couldn't smell a thing, and would certainly sit far away, as would most people, if the truth was otherwise.

Maria also had intrusive thoughts consisting of the single words 'bitch' and 'bastard'. These words often triggered the onset of auditory hallucinations. The therapist and patient made an audiotape with these words repeated over and over. Maria was instructed to listen to this tape in an effort to reduce the anxiety aroused by the words. She was greatly amused while making the tape, and she and the therapist had fits of laughter over it.

These vignettes demonstrate the importance of involving families in the treatment process and highlight the role of behavioral techniques such as exposure in vivo and cognitive restructuring and reframing. The first vignette illustrates that eliciting the reasons for not using coping strategies can uncover complex beliefs. Fiona's story also demonstrates how planning for future events can be important in instilling hope and how the therapist can find concrete ways to demonstrate optimism. The second vignette provides an example of why opportunities to gently challenge beliefs need to be constantly sought and how requesting input from trusted others can be useful. Additionally, the therapist's adoption of an inquisitive and persistent approach, as well as humor, can be an invaluable aide.

Conclusion

It is likely that pharmacological and psychosocial treatments effect different treatment outcomes and that the two treatments may have complex interactions. TREAT is currently overseeing a randomized controlled trial (the Recovery Plus Study) designed to establish the relative and combined effectiveness of the early introduction of STOPP and clozapine. Consecutive first-episode patients who do not achieve a certain level of remission after the initial 12 weeks of treatment are randomly assigned to one of four groups for a further 12 week period: (1) standard antipsychotic therapy; (2) standard antipsychotic therapy and STOPP; (3) clozapine; and (4) clozapine and STOPP. All groups receive case management services. Of the 283 individuals with positive symptoms at 12 weeks identified over the past four years, 88 (31%) were eligible for the trial, and 47 (53%) of those have agreed to participate; the recruitment phase of the study ceased in March 2002.

TREAT was developed to assist in the early identification of people experiencing persisting positive or negative psychotic symptoms after their first or a subsequent acute episode, and to facilitate assertive and systematic intervention. It provides an ongoing clinical resource for case managers and clinicians within EPPIC and in the wider health care network. The monitoring of prolonged recovery in early psychosis through regular and mandatory team review could be applicable y to other mental health services.

Acknowledgements

The Recovery Plus Study is supported by the Victorian Health Promotion Foundation and by Novartis. The authors acknowledge the contributions of Melanie Davern, Debbie Dick, Simone Pica, Richard Bell, Chris Pantelis, Brendan Murphy, Dianne Albiston, and Lorelle Drew in the development of the Treatment Resistance Early Assessment Team, and Susy Harrigan in data analysis.

References

1. McGorry PD, Edwards J, Mihalopoulos C, et al (1996) EPPIC: an evolving system of early detection and optimal management. *Schizophrenia Bulletin* 22:305–326.
2. Edwards J, McGorry P (2002) Implementing Early Intervention in Psychosis: A Guide to Establishing Early Psychosis Services. London, Martin Dunitz.
3. EPPIC: Prolonged Recovery in Early Psychosis (2002) A Treatment Manual and Video. Melbourne, Early Psychosis Prevention and Intervention Centre.
4. Lukoff D, Neuchterlein KH., Ventura J (1986) Manual for the Expanded Brief Psychiatric Rating Scale. *Psychiatric Bulletin* **12**:594–602.
5. Jackson HJ, McGorry, PD, Edwards J (2001) Cognitively oriented psychotherapy for early psychosis: Theory, praxis, outcome, and challenges, in Social Cognition and Schizophrenia, Edited by Corrigan P, Penn D. Washington, DC, APA Press.
6. Herrmann-Doig T, Maude D, Edwards J (2002) Systematic Treatment of Persistent Psychosis (STOPP): A psychological approach to facilitating recovery in young people with first-episode psychosis. London, Martin Dunitz.
7. Wing J, Curtis R, Beevor A (1996) HoNOS: The Health of the Nation Outcome Scales, Report on Research July 1993 - December 1995. London, College Research Unit, Royal College of Psychiatrists.
8. Andreasen, NC (1982) Negative symptoms in schizophrenia: Definitions and reliability. *Archives of General Psychiatry* **39**:784–788.
9. Heinrichs, DW, Hanlon, TE, Carpenter, WT (1994) The quality of life scale: An instrument for rating the schizophrenic deficit syndrome. *Schizophrenia Bulletin* **10**:388–398.

Appendix II
STOPP Discharge Report

Aaron

Introduction to STOPP therapy

STOPP sessions are offered to clients at EPPIC who continue to experience positive symptoms after 3 months of treatment. STOPP therapists provide short-term psychological therapy as an adjunct to routine clinical care. They assess enduring psychotic symptoms, current coping style and premorbid/comorbid contributing factors using a cognitively-orientated framework. The therapy provides psychoeducation, addresses stigma and assists with coping skills. It focuses on strengthening identity and improving self esteem and social functioning, and also on belief modification and cognitive restructuring with regard to psychotic symptoms.

Aaron attended 16 (out of a possible 24) one-hour sessions of STOPP over 12 weeks. He found it difficult to commit to all sessions because of avolition and ambivalence about attendance. The therapist visited Aaron at home on several occasions to promote engagement.

Background summary

Aaron, 19, is unemployed and shares accommodation with two friends. When first assessed at EPPIC, he had a 13-month history of deteriorating function and psychotic symptoms. Positive symptoms included thought disorder and auditory hallucinations (predominately malicious in nature). He experienced hallucinations continuously throughout the day, and referred to the voices as 'telepathy' from other people. The voices sometimes reinforced his thoughts and sometimes offered contradictory opinions which were confusing and distressing. Aaron was worried that people could read his mind. He was anxious, preoccupied with his poor interpersonal relationships, and experienced alogia and disorganisation. Aaron was admitted to the EPPIC inpatient unit in May 2002.

Aaron's parents separated prior to his birth but his mother re-married when he was a toddler. He has two half-siblings (aged 14 and 12 years) from this partnership. He described his relationship with his mother, Jan, and stepfather, Max, as volatile and emotionally abusive. He said that Max was verbally 'malicious' toward him, and that his mother was unwilling to support or protect him in conflicts with Max.

Aaron enjoyed bushwalking and hiking during his secondary school years, and found these activities a way of escaping the intense emotional situation at home. He performed well academically and excelled in artistic expression such as drawing, painting and photography. His few friends at school did not 'fit in' with the rest of his peers.

Aaron met his biological father, Tom, for the first time when he was 17. He then lived and worked with his father for 6 months. However, Tom asked Aaron to leave home due to relationship difficulties between them. Aaron believed Tom was disappointed with him, but never fully understood why he was asked to leave. He has since struggled to support himself financially.

There is no family history of psychotic illness and Aaron denied illicit substance use.

Reason for referral to STOPP

Aaron was referred to STOPP by his case manager because he was struggling to cope with psychotic symptoms after 4 months of treatment at EPPIC. Aaron had been prescribed risperidone and then olanzapine, in addition to an antidepressant, with minimal impact on psychotic symptoms. During this initial period, Aaron's compliance with medication was assessed as 'adequate'. At the point of referral to STOPP Aaron was commenced on clozapine.

Aaron was unwilling to permit his case manager to make contact with his family to inform them of his illness, but allowed him to speak with his housemates to provide psychoeducation and support. Aaron was offered the opportunity to participate in an art therapy program and group excursions, but he declined. The case manager said Aaron was difficult to engage and preoccupied with his auditory hallucinations, and suggested he be considered for STOPP therapy to help alleviate some of the associated distress.

Presenting concerns at STOPP

Aaron was articulate and appeared intelligent, but frequently displayed thought blocking, latency of response and poverty of speech. His thoughts were tangential and it was difficult to engage him in conversation for longer than 30 minutes. He had blunted affect and appeared unkempt.

Aaron said he had problems with lack of energy ('I can't get out of bed in the morning'), repetitive and indecisive thinking and 'telepathic' communications. He often felt he needed to be doing multiple tasks simultaneously, and would frequently engage in internal circular arguments about whether or not to do something.

Aaron identified two telepathic voices, both of whom were unfamiliar and of unspecified gender. They spoke whole sentences, and were sometimes supportive and at other times discouraging or malicious – for example, 'No, that's a dumb idea, don't do that!' He had difficulty concentrating and rated himself as moderately depressed.

Aaron's negative symptoms and guarded presentation made it difficult to elicit information. This was addressed through having briefer meetings, a longer assessment phase, and incorporating additional information obtained during the treatment phases.

Formulation for Psychological Intervention

The working formulation was based on assessment throughout STOPP, including discussions with the case manager and treating doctor.

Predisposing factors

There was no evidence of established risk factors which increase the susceptibility for psychosis such as obstetric complications, other brain insults or a family history of schizophrenia. However, temperament and personality can influence the content of psychosis, interact with the response to psychosis and related stressors, and possibly (although more speculative) contribute to factors which result in the expression of a vulnerability to psychosis.

Aaron described a sense of insecurity and abandonment arising from the turbulent relationship with his mother and step-father and lack of contact with his biological father. He frequently perceived situations as either good or bad, and had a tendency to idealise relationships. He then condemned others and himself when the relationships did not meet his expectations, and was fearful of investing in relationships in case they failed.

Precipitating factors

Aaron's acute psychotic symptoms were preceded by a 12-month period of financial problems and emotional uncertainty with regard to his family. Difficulties in establishing a relationship with his father may have added to his feelings of rejection and loss. Aaron expressed an overwhelming impression that he had been unable to meet the expectations of his parents. Recent confusion over his sexual preferences and the failure of several relationships with females had compounded these 'painful' experiences and led him to question his self-worth and identity. The additional demands of changing accommodation added significant stress.

Perpetuating factors

Aaron's inconsistent use of prescribed medication (revealed during STOPP sessions) compromised response to pharmacological treatment, delaying recovery and exacerbating his social and emotional difficulties.

Aaron's negative cognitive assumptions about himself and others, combined with a lack of energy and flattened mood, perpetuated his relationship difficulties. He became confused and distressed when the voices offered comments that contradicted his own thoughts. The voices increased in intensity when under emotional strain, which usually involved interpersonal relationships. Aaron was aware of the toll his relationships had taken on his emotional and mental well-being. He seemed to protect himself from emotional investment by procrastinating about initiating social contact or engaging in shared activity. His negative symptoms and depressed mood increased his tendency to avoid socialisation. Although the stress associated with interpersonal interactions may have weakened Aaron's capacity to recover from psychosis, participation in pleasurable activities could have helped to boost his self-confidence, lift his mood, and lessen his preoccupation with psychotic symptoms.

Impact of psychosis

Aaron felt he had failed in his attempts to embark on a career. He had a natural inclination toward the arts, but seemed not to value these abilities as worthwhile occupational pursuits. He had also experienced great difficulty in finding work in this area. Aaron was very conscious of others' disappointment in him, and his own disappointment with himself, and expressed anger about not having made something of himself and his opportunities. These frustrations were heightened by his psychotic symptoms, which reduced his capacity for goal-directed activity.

Psychological interventions to date

Since Aaron did not attend 24 sessions of STOPP, progress through all phases of the therapy was compromised. However, he appeared to have obtained some benefit from the intervention.

Developing a collaborative working relationship

Aaron was reluctant to discuss the nature of his symptoms and consider explanations for his experiences. Initially he feared sharing details about his telepathic experiences, as he was uncertain whether the voices would object. He was more willing to explore precipitating and perpetuating stressors associated with his confused thinking, particularly as it related to interpersonal relationships, so this issue was established as the first item on the agenda for therapy. Discussion regarding his relationships enabled later exploration of the meaning of his symptoms, and some collaborative reality testing of his telepathic experiences.

Aaron spent considerable time discussing the grief he experienced from his difficult and disappointing relationships with his parents. He now recognises that he has developed some unhelpful beliefs about himself and others' intentions, and that these beliefs affect his self-esteem and relationships with others.

Exploring and coping with psychosis

Aaron was reluctant to talk about psychosis so it was difficult to provide psychoeducation about the illness. However, during discussion of his ambivalence about attending treatment sessions, he acknowledged he had been inconsistent in taking his medication. He appeared to be unconvinced of the need to take antipsychotics, despite education from his case manager as to its importance. This was explored further, and he acknowledged experiencing troublesome side-effects. Aaron was encouraged to discuss this concern with his treating doctor who reassessed and adjusted his medication, leading to improvements in his function and compliance.

Aaron made a concerted effort to listen to pacifying voices rather than those that were derogatory or malicious. When derogatory voices interfered with decision making, he found it helpful to silently repeat the word 'STOP' to himself and use distraction. He was then able to think more clearly and re-direct his attention to the task at hand. Aaron has also learned to ignore unconstructive voices by listening to relaxation music through headphones, humming to himself, or talking to his housemates.

Aaron has considered the idea that the conflicting points of view expressed by the voices mirror his own thought processes, but he is unclear as to how or why the telepathic opinions could be so similar to his own thoughts. He has been encouraged to consider how people may be able to insert thoughts, opinions, and ideas into his mind, and to think of ways to test whether people could telepathically receive his thoughts. In a meeting with his treating doctor, and another psychiatrist for a second opinion, he discussed research on these unusual experiences. Both doctors suggested that sometimes people could mistake their own thoughts for those of other people who had expressed similar ideas. Aaron felt this explanation was somewhat convincing, and now wishes to reconsider whether this might be the case for him. More work is required to assist Aaron to reflect on how he can understand his hallucinations.

Aaron has started working toward two goals – learning rock climbing and building relationships – but has been frustrated with the slow progress. Nevertheless, he feels he is enjoying life more than before.

Strengthening the capacity to relate to others

Aaron has become increasingly aware of his 'black and white' thinking about himself and others. He understands this behaviour as a 'survival' mechanism to help him concentrate on good experiences. However, he also recognises that this strategy is problematic because it makes him think in extremes. During therapy, Aaron was encouraged to consider both the positive and less desirable aspects of situations at the same time, and has found this a useful exercise. He has also been encouraged to challenge some of his negative thoughts and has had some success. He reports feeling better about himself, and has an improved mood, when he successfully challenges negative assumptions.

Response to therapy

Despite the difficulties in engaging Aaron, he has shown an ability to explore sensitive grief and loss issues in a therapeutic setting, trial some coping strategies, and consider alternative reasons for some of his psychotic experiences (for example, that his telepathic experiences may be misattributions of his own thoughts). Aaron's general functioning has improved, and if he works further on the areas addressed and consistently takes his medication, he should continue to make progress.

Recommendations to the case manager

- Flexibly adjust the frequency of appointments, provide assertive follow-up for failed attendance, and remain aware that Aaron's ambivalence about relationships may affect the treatment process.
- Closely monitor Aaron's depressive symptoms and compliance with medication.
- Continue to sensitively approach psychoeducation about psychosis. Aaron needs further help to understand the reasons for his confused thinking, lack of energy, and 'telepathic' experiences.
- Provide realistic expectations about the expected slow pace of recovery.
- Consider the use of guided reality testing to help challenge Aaron's beliefs that others can read his mind or send telepathic messages to him.
- Provide an ongoing cognitively-oriented focus to help Aaron recognise extremes in his thinking and to balance this with more realistic views about self and others. Focus particularly on his tendency to catastrophise interpersonal events and overestimate his own shortcomings.
- Help Aaron to link the emotional distress arising from his unhelpful assumptions about himself and others with an increase in psychotic symptoms.
- Work toward goals that help Aaron to feel good about himself and recognise his capacities and his achievements. In particular, maintain a focus on long-term vocational and socialisation goals.

Index

A

activity scheduling 41

adolescence, psychotic disorders 2–3, 9–10, 13–18

agenda, collaborative 29–31

Antecedent and Coping Interview 21

anxiety, comorbid with psychosis 8, 37

assessment

  case example 26–7

  cognitive-behavioural framework 21–3

  instruments 20–1

  personal and family history 24–5

  trauma 23–4

Australian Clinical Guidelines for Early Psychosis 1

B

Beck Depression Inventory II 21

beliefs 24, 35, 57–8

  reality testing 44–5

Beliefs About Voices Questionnaire 21

Brief Psychiatric Rating Scale, 24-item 20–1

C

cannabis misuse, in psychotic disorders 3–4
clinical service 5
closure, therapeutic relationship 17, 63–71
cognitive-behavioural framework, in assessment 21–3
cognitive-behavioural therapy
  evaluation 5–6, 7–9
  limitations 9
collaborative working relationship 19–32
  agenda 29–31
  assessment 20–7
  difficulties 20
  psychological formulation 27–9
coping skills
  assessment 38–40
  assessment instruments 21
coping strategies
  difficulties using 34–6
  distraction therapy 41
  exposure therapy 42–3
  introducing 40–1
  life skills 45–6
  reality testing 44–5
Coping Strategies List 21

D

delusions
  assessment instruments 21
  coping strategies 41
depression
  assessment instruments 21
  comorbid with psychosis 8, 37
development, effect of psychotic disorders 2–3, 9–10, 24–5, 56
  see also identity, sense of
disapppointment, closing therapeutic relationship 66–7
distraction therapy 41

E

early intervention 2, 4
Early Psychosis Prevention and Intervention Centre (EPICC) 1
emotional responses
  assessment 22
  coping skills 38–45
engagement, in therapeutic relationship 12, 13–18, 65
EPICC (Early Psychosis Prevention and Intervention Centre) 1
erotomania, case example 60
exposure therapy 41, 42–3

F

family history, assessment 24–5
family therapy 25, 66
finishing, therapeutic relationship 17, 63–71
focusing therapy 41, 42–3
formulation, psychological 27–9
future, planning 68

G

Global Scale of Delusional Severity 21
goals 29–30, 68

H

hallucinations, coping strategies 41
hand-over, therapeutic relationship 69–70

I

identity, sense of 10, 11, 24, 52, 54–5, 56–8
  see also development, effect of psychotic disorders
integration 51–61
intervention, early 2, 4

K

Knowledge of Psychosis Questionnaire 21

L

life issues 45–6, 54–5
loss and disappointment, therapeutic relationship 66–7

M

Maudsley Assessment for Delusions Schedule 21
medication, non-compliance 37
motivational interviewing techniques 37

P

paranoia, case example 57–8
personal history, assessment 24–5, 56
planning 68
posttraumatic stress disorder 23–4
prolonged recovery 5–6, 11–12, 24, 35, 45–6
psychoeducation 30, 34, 36, 49
psychological formulation 27–9
psychopathology, assessment instruments 20–1
psychotic disorders
  in adolescence 2–3, 9–10, 13–18
  biological intervention 4
  coping skills 38–40
  coping strategies 34–6, 40–5
  early intervention 2
  exploring 33–8
  psychological intervention 4–6, 7–12
  social intervention 4
  in young people 2–3, 9–10, 13–18
Psychotic Symptom Rating Scales 21
psychotic symptoms
  assessment instruments 21
  cognitive-behavioural therapy 5–6
  coping skills 38–40
  coping strategies 34–6, 40–5
  meaning of 58–61
  negative 10–11

R

reality testing 8, 44–5
recovery, prolonged 5–6, 11–12, 24, 35, 45–6
Recovery Plus Project 5, 6
relapse prevention 68–9
relationship, therapeutic *see* therapeutic relationship
relationships, personal 24–5, 51–61
Revised Beck Depression Inventory 21

S

Scale for the Assessment of Negative Symptoms 21
self, sense of 10, 11, 24, 52, 54–5, 56–8
  see also development, effect of psychotic disorders
self-exploration 53–4
self-expression 52–3
social links 67–8
STOPP *see* Systematic Treatment of Persistent Psychosis
substance misuse, in psychotic disorders 3–4
support network 65–6, 67–8
Systematic Treatment of Persistent Psychosis (STOPP) 1–2
  engagement 13–18
  evaluation 5–6
  phases 11–12, 13–18

T

tension, reducing 41
therapeutic process 13–18
therapeutic relationship
  closing 17, 63–71
  engagement 13–18
trauma, assessment 23–4
TREAT (Treatment Resistant Early Assessment Team) 2, 79, 84
treatment goals 29–30, 68
Treatment Resistant Early Assessment (TREAT) 1–2
24-item Brief Psychiatric Rating Scale 20–1

Y

young people, psychotic disorders 2–3, 9–10, 13–18